RELIEVING SCIATICA

Larry P. Credit, OMD
Sharon G. Hartunian, LICSW
Margaret J. Nowak, CMT

AVERY PUBLISHING GROUP
Garden City Park • New York

The publisher does not advocate the use of any particular form of health care but believes the information presented in this book should be available to the public. Because each person and situation are unique, the authors and publisher urge the reader to check with a qualified health professional before using a procedure for which there is any question of appropriateness. Treatments always involve some risk; therefore, the authors and publisher disclaim responsibility for any ill effects or harmful consequences resulting from the use of the approaches discussed in this book.

This text is as timely and accurate as its publisher and authors can make it. All listed addresses, phone numbers, websites, etc. have been reviewed and updated during the production process. However, the data is subject to change. Refer to other current sources of information to verify textual material.

Cover Design: Phaedra Mastrocola and
      Eric Macaluso
In-House Editor: Helene Ciaravino
Typesetter: Gary A. Rosenberg
Printer: Paragon Press, Honesdale, PA

Avery Publishing Group
120 Old Broadway
Garden City Park, NY 11040
1–800–548–5757
www.averypublishing.com

Library of Congress Cataloging-in-Publication Data

Credit, Larry, P.
    Relieving sciatica : using complementary medicine to overcome the
pain of sciatica / by Larry P. Credit, Sharon G. Hartunian, Margaret
J. Nowak.
    p. cm.
    Includes bibliographic references and index.
    ISBN 0–89529–921–6
    1. Sciatica Popular works. 2. Sciatica—Alternative treatment
Popular works. I. Hartunian, Sharon G. II. Nowak, Margaret J.
III. Title
RC420.C74 2000
616.8′7—dc21   99–32978
                                                      CIP

Printed in the United States of America

10 9 8 7 6 5 4 3 2 1

Contents

Acknowledgments, vii

Preface, ix

PART I   SCIATICA: SYMPTOMS AND SOLUTIONS

Introduction, 1

Defining Sciatica, 3

Treating Sciatica, 15

Conclusion, 23

PART II   TREATMENT APPROACHES

Introduction, 25

Acupressure, 27

Acupuncture, 30

Alexander Technique, 34

Aquatic Therapy, 38

Chiropractic, 42

Emotional Pain Relief
   Therapy, 46

Feldenkrais Method, 55

Foot Reflexology, 58

Hatha Yoga, 61

Massage, 65

Myotherapy, 71

Nutritional Counseling, 75

Osteopathy, 80

Personal Training, 84

Qigong, 90

Relaxation/Meditation, 93

Rolfing, 101

Tai Chi, 105

Trager Approach, 108

Conclusion, 113

Glossary, 115

Research Issues, 117

Health Insurance Issues, 121

Notes, 125

Index, 131

We dedicate our second book to our parents and our children.
The wisdom and love of our parents enables us to strive
towards a legacy of honor for Talyn, Sara, and Cali.

Acknowledgments

We are fully appreciative of the editing expertise of Helene Ciaravino and the guidance of Rudy Shur in the publication of our second book on complementary medicine. Helene, you are a joy to work with and a trusted sage with the English language. Rudy, you continue to display the foresight needed to mold a book's vision into a practical reality. To our colleagues in the field of integrative medicine, we applaud you in your efforts to secure a healthier future.

Preface

The statistics on the prevalence of low back pain and its economic consequences are astounding. Consider, for example, the following facts:

- Low back pain affects 60 to 90 percent of the world population over the life span.[1, 2]

- The cost of care for low back pain in the United States, covering medical care, worker's compensation payments, and time lost from work, has been estimated to be $50 billion annually.[3]

- The economic costs to patients in the United States is at least $16 billion every year.[4]

- Back problems are cited as the most frequent cause of activity impairment in people less than 45 years of age, affecting 5.4 million Americans each year.[5, 6]

- Present day estimates indicate that eight out of ten American adults will experience low back problems during the course of their lifetimes.[7]

This high incidence of low back problems results in extensive physical and emotional suffering for many individuals. Quite a few of these cases involve sciatica.

Sciatica is a painful symptom under the category of low back pain. The pain of sciatica is felt along the course of the sciatic nerve, which runs from the low back into the buttock area, down the back of the thigh and the inner leg, and extends as far down as the foot. The pain can begin abruptly or can develop gradually. It has been described as a severe, sharp, electrical pain with burning and aching components. Each year, about 5 percent of the general population will experience sciatica, with lifetime prevalence being 40 percent.[8] This book aims to inform the reader of the various complementary care treatment options that may ease the symptoms of sciatica, decrease the time of the recovery period, and prevent further flare-ups. Our goal is to provide hope and guidance for those suffering from this condition.

Part 1 of *Relieving Sciatica* defines sciatica, discusses its symptoms, and gives an overview of the thought behind both conventional and alternative approaches to its treatment. Part II offers detailed information on over fifteen complementary medicine options. For each option, we provide straightforward details on the approach itself; how it views and treats sciatica, in particular; relevant research, if applicable; estimated cost and duration; health insurance coverage information; the credentials and education to look for in a practitioner; and a helpful source through which further information is available. Where possible, useful at-home techniques are described, and dispersed throughout the book are tips for pain relief, from positioning to soaking to exercising. A glossary serves as a handy quick reference tool, and the back of the book has up-to-date reports on current research and health insurance issues.

If you or someone you love suffers from sciatica, there is something you can do about it. *Relieving Sciatica* will help you to understand the pain, to find the best treatment, and to become a more effective healthcare consumer.

PART I

Sciatica: Symptoms and Solutions

The term *sciatica* may seem technical and confusing. What's real is the pain. The first step in easing your discomfort is to learn the basics of sciatica—a condition from which so few sufferers have found avenues of relief. Part I answers the following common questions: What triggers sciatica? What is the range of symptoms? How has sciatica been managed conventionally? Can complementary medicine provide the relief that conventional medicine has not aptly provided? In the following pages, we cover everything from symptoms to solutions, and we offer important guidance for getting started on a plan that works for you.

Defining Sciatica

Y ou may have been diagnosed with sciatica, or you may suspect that you have it. Either way, the name of the condition is
intimidating, and so is the pain. This section will explain what
sciatica is, discuss its symptoms, and describe possible causes.

WHAT IS SCIATICA?

Sciatica is an irritation or compression of the sciatic nerve. To understand how and why this condition occurs, it is first necessary to learn
the very basic anatomy of the spine. The spinal area includes: the
spinal cord, made up of nerves; the vertebrae; the intervertebral
discs; the muscles; the tendons; the ligaments; and the connective
tissues.

Nerves allow communication throughout the body. The bundle of
nerves that make up the *spinal cord* travels from the brain through the
entire length of the spinal canal, and small groups of these nerves
branch off to various parts of the body. The *vertebrae* are an interlocking series of nearly circular-shaped bones of differing sizes. Each
vertebra has a hole in the middle through which the spinal cord runs.
There are twenty-four vertebrae, divided into three sections: the
seven cervical vertebrae; the twelve thoracic vertebrae; and the five
lumbar vertebrae. These bones provide support and protection for
the spinal cord, and allow the back to twist and move in numerous
ways. The *intervertebral discs,* composed of cartilage, separate the vertebrae and cushion them during movement. At the end of the spinal
cord is the *sacrum,* which is a triangular-shaped bone plate formed
from five fused vertebrae, and finally the tiny *coccyx,* also a triangular-shaped bone, formed from several rudimentary vertebrae. See
Figures 1.1 and 1.2 for an illustration of these components of the
spinal area.

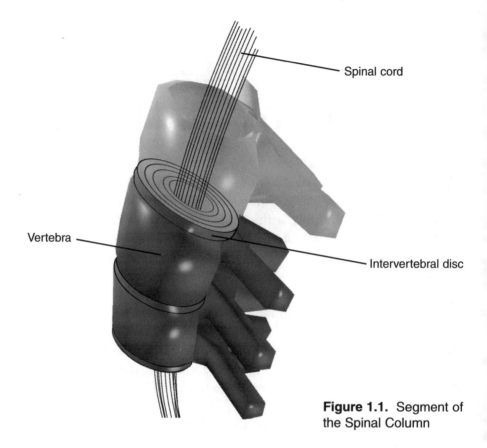

Spinal cord

Vertebra

Intervertebral disc

Figure 1.1. Segment of the Spinal Column

The *muscles* in the back support the spine in an upright position and also allow the back to rotate, twist, bend, and maintain proper spinal curves. *Tendons* connect muscles to bones, allowing the contracted muscles to move the bones smoothly. *Ligaments* connect bones to bones, providing support and proper movement of joints. Finally, the *connective tissue* supports, binds, and connects body structures. Obviously, when healthy, all of these components work together to allow you easy movement and considerable flexibility.

When viewing a person's spine from the back of the body, the vertebrae appear to form a straight column of interlocking bones. This is evident in Figure 1.2 (page 5). But the view from the side of the body, as depicted in Figure 1.3 (page 6), reveals three natural, spinal curves: one in the neck; another in the upper back; and the third in the low back region. (This, of course, does not include the very end of the spinal column; there are natural curves in the coccyx

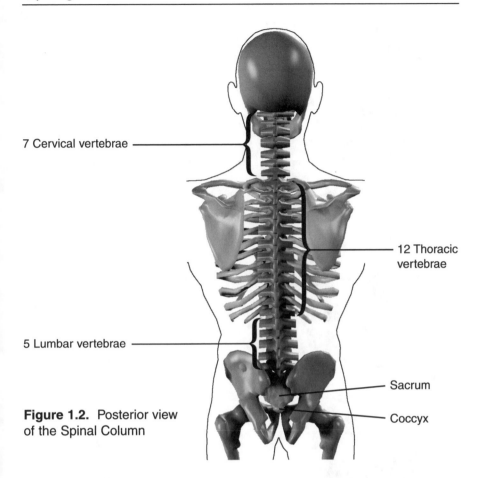

7 Cervical vertebrae

12 Thoracic vertebrae

5 Lumbar vertebrae

Sacrum

Coccyx

Figure 1.2. Posterior view of the Spinal Column

area, as well.) These three curves indicate a flexible structure with the ability for give and take. All components of the spine and back rely on each other for the entire spinal system to function properly. A problem in one area can have a consequent negative impact on another.

The *sciatic nerve* is formed from several spinal nerves that pass through the openings in the sacrum—as mentioned previously, the lower portion of the spine. This nerve is the primary nerve in the leg, and the longest and largest nerve in the body. Its pathway originates in the low back, passes through the deep layers of the buttock muscle, to the back of the thigh, where slightly above the knee it divides into two large branches. The shorter branch of the nerve turns toward the outer edge of the leg and ends just below the kneecap, and the longer branch extends down the back of the leg to the heel area. See

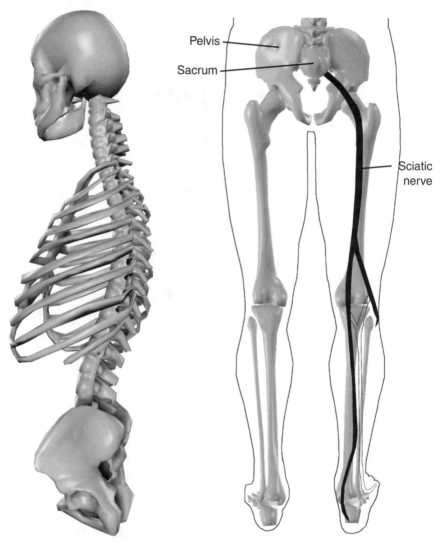

Figure 1.3. Sideview of
the Spinal Column

Figure 1.4. Pathway of the Sciatic
Nerve

Figure 1.4 above for an illustration of this path. When this nerve
is pressed or irritated, a sharp, electrical wave of pain, along with
other symptoms, such as numbness, tingling, weakness, achiness,
and burning, can occur anywhere along the pathway. This is sciatica.

Sciatica is a symptom of and a frequent companion to low back
pain. It can also be a separate problem in and of itself, with its own
symptoms. Although incorrectly thought of as a disease or illness,

sciatica is an inflammatory condition caused, as mentioned above, by irritation or compression of the sciatic nerve. It can be due to a number of possible causes (see below to page 13).

WHAT ARE THE SYMPTOMS OF SCIATICA?

When the sciatic nerve is irritated or compressed by any number of different conditions, aggravating pain can be felt along the nerve pathway. The pain can be constant or intermittent, sudden or progressive. It is characterized by pain radiating down the back of the thigh that has been described as sharp, stabbing, electrical, and burning.

These symptoms can manifest in one or both legs. The pain may be distributed uniformly along the pathway but, often, specific and intense spots of pain are predominant. In many cases, the pain of sciatica is accompanied by sensations of numbness, tingling, weakness, and achiness.

Generally, the sharp, stabbing pain comes on suddenly, reaches a high intensity, then gradually fades away. The burning sensation, which suggests a pinched nerve, is often felt anywhere on the lower back, buttocks, legs, and/or feet. The electrical sensation usually radiates pain from the specific area where the nerve is compressed and, from there, down the sciatic nerve pathway. It comes on suddenly, then disappears, only to return and repeat the cycle. The tingling and numbness are further indications of nerve irritation along the pathway. Finally, the achiness is associated with strained or overworked muscles. The symptoms of sciatica can be more severe when the individual bends forward, coughs, or sneezes.

WHAT ARE THE CAUSES OF SCIATICA?

The sciatic nerve can be irritated by a number of conditions. The most common are: an inflamed piriformis muscle; a herniated lumbar disc; lumbosacral muscle strain; spinal stenosis; a ruptured disc; and emotional stress. Less common causes to consider are: arthritis; endometrial cysts; ankylosing spondylitis; a sacroiliac ligament tear; and weak abdominal and back muscles. These terms may sound overwhelming, but each one is clearly defined within the next couple of pages.

Piriformis Syndrome

The piriformis muscles, which are in the buttock region just above the sciatic nerve, are responsible for rotating the hip outward when standing and for rotating the hip inward when sitting. These muscles can become inflamed from overwork or injury. The inflamed piriformis muscle, in one or both buttocks, can press against the sciatic nerve and therefore cause painful sciatica.

Prime candidates for piriformis syndrome include individuals who sit for extended periods of time, such as car drivers and office workers (especially those who keep their thick wallets in their back pockets), and individuals who stand for long periods of time, playing golf, shoveling snow, etc. Also, people who suffer from accidents that involve falling onto the buttocks, too much aerobic exercise, and simple leg-length discrepancies are at heightened risk for piriformis syndrome.

The primary symptom of piriformis syndrome is tenderness and sudden pain in the buttock region, aggravated by sitting and especially after first getting up in the morning. The discomfort can also follow along the pathway of the sciatic nerve. A tingling, numbing sensation can develop in the buttock and leg region when sitting. The appropriate evaluation for piriformis syndrome would include: a history of injury; the location of pain; assessment of muscle strengths and weaknesses; testing of reflexes; and a musculoskeletal examination.

According to researcher Barton, it has been observed that in some people, the sciatic nerve actually passes through the belly of the piriformis muscle. Anyone with this anatomical condition is more susceptible to developing the symptoms of sciatica. This is due to the fact that the sciatic nerve is more likely to be compressed when the piriformis muscles experience any irritation.[1]

Lumbar Herniated Disc

Lumbar discs are thick cushions of cartilage that separate the vertebrae in the lumbar region of the spine. Each disc has a hard, fibrous outer edge and a soft, gelatin-like substance in the center. They allow greater movement and flexibility between the vertebra and act like shock absorbers, distributing the body's weight when the spine bends. The lumbar discs have no blood supply of their own. Therefore, they absorb nourishment from the surrounding tissue like a sponge.

During cycles of physical activity and rest, the discs squeeze the fluids back to the surrounding tissue and soak up fresh fluids. Over a long process of wearing down, various factors—such as repetitive lifting, poor posture, or loss of flexibility—can inhibit nourishment absorption and cause a disc to become thin and brittle. This leads to a herniated disc.

A herniated disc occurs when some portion of the disc protrudes through the defected, worn-down area. It is a displacement from proper alignment. A symptom of a herniated lumbar disc is a sudden, sharp, electric pain that radiates to the buttock and down the pathway of the sciatic nerve. Secondary symptoms include: stiffness in the lower back; limitation in the flexion and extension of the back; weakened reflexes; numbness; tingling; hot and cold sensations; and hypersensitivity. Coughing and sneezing may aggravate a herniated disc. Standing or lying on the unaffected side and flexing the knees can alleviate it.

Several types of physical assessment may be used to determine a herniated lumber disc. The location of pain, a reflex evaluation, a muscle weakness test, and a sensory loss evaluation of the leg can help diagnose the problem. So, too, can the determination of flexibility in the spine, as well as the performance of a straight-leg-raising test. When a person with a herniated disc has his or her leg raised and straightened, pain will be felt in the leg, not in the back.

Lumbosacral Muscle Strain

When unnecessary tension is placed upon the supporting muscles of the back, strain is placed on the low back—that is, the lumbosacral region. A sedentary lifestyle, obesity, poor posture, and lack of exercise are all contributing factors to lumbosacral problems. A lumbosacral strain usually occurs from lifting objects improperly, from twisting without stretching, or from trauma to the lower back.

Symptoms of lumbosacral muscle strain generally include: the onset of pain after physical activity involving the low back; a dull, aching, persistent pain; and stiffness in the lumbosacral region. When tight muscles in this region press against and irritate the sciatic nerve, a burning, stabbing pain accompanied by some numbness and weakness may occur along the sciatic pathway. The pain radiates across the low back and occasionally into the buttock region. Movement of any kind, particularly standing, lifting, bending, and/or twisting, can aggravate this condition. Sitting and resting may temporarily alleviate it.

Although the strain can go away by itself, if the pain is persistent, a person may decide to seek diagnostic testing. A test to determine lumbosacral muscle strain is the straight-leg-raising test. If there is lumbosacral muscle strain, any pain elicited from this test will be felt in the low back and not in the leg.

Spinal Stenosis

Spinal stenosis is a narrowing of the spinal canal. It is generally seen in the senior population. The narrowing is a result of the formation of bone spurs on the spine. This condition can cause the sciatic nerve to be compressed as it passes through the narrowed canal. There is a gradual onset of pain in the lumber region. The pain may radiate into the buttocks and occasionally down the legs.

The pain of spinal stenosis is brought on with exercise, prolonged standing, walking, or climbing stairs. People who suffer from this condition tire easily and need to rest after traveling short distances because of the back pain. Sometimes the discomfort can be relieved through rest or sitting. A full medical history and physical exam are generally needed to diagnose spinal stenosis.

Ruptured Disc

As explained previously, intervertebral discs are thick cushions of cartilage that separate and support the vertebrae. Often, poor posture will change the alignment of the spine, as it puts continuous strain on the vertebrae and discs. Continued strain over a long period of time can cause a disc to wear down and to protrude through the area of deterioration (herniated disc, see page 8), the outer portion to split, and the disc to rupture—that is, the soft, inner layer of the disc leaks out. A sudden, violent injury may also cause a disc to rupture.

When a disc's fluid leaks out of its encasement, the disc is deprived of any nourishment. As a result, the soft substance slowly dries and is eventually reabsorbed by the body. Before reabsorption

---

Gene Research

*Cutting-edge research in genetics is now finding that a mutant gene may be responsible for sciataca in about 5 percent of sufferers, as reported in the journal **Science**, July, 1999. If this mutation is identified in an individual, he or she can take special measures to avoid factors that may further increase the risk of sciatica. In another study, as yet unpublished, a more common gene has been found that may affect the structural integrity of the intervertebral disc, increasing pressure on the sciatic nerve. Detailed information on the link between genetics and sciatica is just beginning to be documented and published, but within the near future, strides in this research area are likely to be made.[2]*

---

can occur, the presence of this gelatin-like substance can cause inflammation and swelling in the surrounding area. Radiating pain can be triggered down the thigh and lower leg when any part of the protruding disc presses against the sciatic nerve.

An evaluation to determine the presence of a ruptured disc may include: a full medical history; determination of the precise location of pain and the type of pain; a reflex assessment; and tests for muscle weakness and sensory loss, particularly in the leg region experiencing sciatic symptoms. A person with a ruptured disc will experience limitations in performing the straight-leg-raising test due to pain and/or lack of flexibility. Coughing, sneezing, and/or straining can aggravate a ruptured disc.

Emotional Stress

Emotional stress can be either a direct cause or a contributing factor to low back pain. Stress often occurs when the continuous demands of life overwhelm our ability to cope with them. These demands—stressors—can be internal, involving emotions and attitudes. They can also be external, involving events in our lives that we cannot control, such as traffic and work deadlines. The body reacts to stressors by releasing stress hormones that increase heart rate and breathing rate, as well as tighten muscles throughout the body.

Physical activity (running, walking, movement of some kind) will dissipate stress hormones. When a physical response is not taken, the body remains in a constant state of alert. As a result, physical symptoms can develop, such as backache, fatigue, insomnia, loss of appetite, or the desire to overeat. Emotional symptoms can also develop, such as increased tension, anger, anxiety, and the inability to concentrate, which further complicate the stressful situation and perpetuate the problem.

Sciatica can be a side effect of stress. Contraction of muscles in response to stress can cause back problems and associated symptoms, including sciatica. Measures should be taken to bring relaxation to the muscles. These can involve physical approaches, such as massage and the application of heat, and mental approaches such as meditation.

Arthritis

Arthritis can be the culprit when it comes to sciatica, although it's not a common cause. Arthritis is the term used for the inflammation of a joint and the consequent symptoms of pain, swelling, and changes in the structure of the body. Such changes could include deterioration of cartilage (a dense connective tissue that cushions parts of the skeleton), the overgrowth of bone, and the impairment of function.

Osteoarthritis, also known as degenerative arthritis, is a common form of joint disease, a chronic disability, and a gradual consequence of aging. During the aging process, cartilage deteriorates and places stress on the joints. Symptoms of osteoarthritis include: intensifying pain in the joints; stiffness; mobility limitations; and deformities. If osteoarthritis affects the spinal area, pain can be felt in the low back or down the legs.

Rheumatoid arthritis is a chronic inflammatory disease that can severely effect the joints and the structures of the body, resulting in crippling deformities. It is less common than osteoarthritis. Knees, hips, hands, wrists, elbows, and feet are affected, and there is eventual deterioration in the spinal area. The exact cause is unknown; although, for the most part, it is considered an autoimmune disorder, in which the body's immune system mistakenly attacks its own tissues. Generally, initial onset occurs during middle age.

Sciatica can be caused by either of the above-described types of arthritis, as inflammation, inflexibility, and changes in bones/joints occur. The sciatic nerve may be compressed as its pathway is distorted or obstructed by the effects of arthritis on the spinal column.

Endometrial Cysts

Endometriosis is a painful disease in which tissue that is identical to that in the uterus grows in other parts of the body. This abnormal tissue is often referred to as nodules, cysts, scar tissue, and/or lesions. Such growth can occur in various areas. When the growth of endometrial tissue occurs in the pelvic region, it can lead to sciatica, particularly during menstrual periods when this tissue can engorge and shed, causing bleeding. If you suspect that you may have this condition, it is important to consult a gynecologist, who can investigate the problem.

Ankylosing Spondylitis

Spondylitis refers to an inflammation in the vertebrae; ankylosis refers to the immobility of a joint. Therefore, ankylosing spondylitis indicates both an inflammation and immobility/stiffness of the spine; it is considered an arthritic disorder. The pain and inflammation can start in the low back and work up the spine. Ankylosing spondylitis can begin affecting an individual at 20 years of age, with a gradual worsening of symptoms over time. As deterioration occurs in the cartilage of the intervertebral discs, the body goes through a healing process and scar tissue forms. The scar tissue eventually becomes bone and, as a result, the vertebrae fuse.

Pain and stiffness caused by ankylosing spondylitis vary from person to person, from minimal pain and stiffness to severe, ongoing pain and deformities of the spine. The specific cause of this condition is not known, but it is generally considered to be an autoimmune disorder, in which the immune system of the body mistakenly attacks its own tissue. Symptoms of sciatic nerve irritation can be experienced during the early stages of ankylosing spondylitis, but sciatica is not specifically used as a sign of early diagnosis for the disease.

Sacroiliac Ligament Tear

The sacroiliac ligaments hold the hip bones to the sacrum, helping to stabilize the back of the pelvic region. When injury to these ligaments occurs, pain is felt across the lower back and down the thigh. This pain may be due, in part, to sciatica, as swelling from the injury may result in a compressed sciatic nerve.

Weak Muscles

A sedentary lifestyle (including a lack of exercise), excess weight gain, and poor posture can all cause weakness of the musculature that supports the spine. When the muscles of the abdomen and the supporting muscles of the back are weak, they cannot adequately hold the spine erect. This leaves nerves vulnerable to pinching. The sciatic nerve is particularly susceptible to pressure that results from inadequate positioning of the spine.

It is clear that there are a number of conditions—some chronic, some acute—that can result in sciatica. It is best to seek the diagnosis of a healthcare professional, so that you can identify the specific disorder and benefit from any available treatments. The following section discusses the treatments traditionally used by conventional medicine, as well as the philosophies behind complementary medicine's more *holistic* approach—considering the whole person, including physical, emotional, mental, spiritual, social, and environmental aspects. However, it will become clear that both conventional and complementary medicine are compatible with each other, and that the future of health care is moving in that very direction.

Treating Sciatica

The causes of sciatica are numerous, and each individual who experiences the condition may have a number of factors contributing to his or her pain. As a result, treatment protocols will vary. In most cases, optimal relief is achieved through a combination of treatments that spans the following: specific therapeutic approaches, including both conventional and complementary techniques; a modification in the activities of daily living that contribute to the condition; and stress management and/or relaxation. Similar to putting out a raging fire, the best way to smother the flames of sciatic pain is to surround the condition with treatment elements that will subdue the escalation of pain and set the stage for the rebuilding and healing process.

As suggested in the information above, modern health care can categorize a given treatment under one of two categories: conventional medicine or complementary medicine. The following section briefly discusses the concepts behind these general labels.

CONVENTIONAL MEDICINE'S APPROACH

The conventional medical approach to the treatment of sciatica presently embraces the philosophy that a number of techniques used together in a comprehensive program will bring the greatest relief for the individual.[1, 2, 3] Prior to this multifaceted approach, the traditional recommendations were long-term bed rest, narcotic pain medication, and surgery. These have been replaced, for the most part, by short-term bed rest, nonsteroidal anti-inflammatory medication (NSAIDs), the continuation of reasonable daily activities, and rehabilitation approaches that may involve gentle stretching, massage, physical therapy, chiropractic treatments, and stress management/relaxation.

This present trend encompasses approaches and ideas embraced by complementary medicine. In addition to incorporating the complementary approaches of massage, chiropractic, and relaxation techniques, the conventional approach is addressing the uniqueness of back pain for each individual. Along with a routine medical history, conventional practitioners are increasingly taking into account a person's present life situation, along with his or her work and activity habits, to assess the connection between lifestyle and the symptoms of low back pain. Conventional medicine is also moving toward avoiding costly and unnecessary invasive treatments in treating low back problems. Of course, there are cases for which surgery is strongly suggested.

In the following paragraphs, we will review some of the traditionally used treatments for sciatica. Included are descriptions of commonly prescribed medications, physical therapy, surgery, and a few other mainstream approaches. The type of treatment recommended is generally directed by the cause of the symptoms.

Medication

There are various types of medicines used in the treatment of sciatica. Some are taken orally, while others are injected. Orally administered medications may serve a number of goals. Nonsteroidal anti-inflammatory drugs (NSAIDs) reduce swelling in muscles and decrease the pain caused by this inflammation. Narcotic pain medication simply decreases pain. Muscle relaxants tranquilize muscles and relax spasms. Sedatives decrease anxiety.

People with very localized pain may prefer injections that begin working immediately on the specific problem areas. Steroid injections and local anesthetics decrease inflammation and relieve tension in tight muscles. Trigger point injections, which deliver a procaine-saline solution directly into the painful trigger point of the muscle, enable the muscle to relax and stretch out.

Physical Therapy

Physical therapy is a general term that covers many forms of treatment. Some of these are quite helpful in relieving the pain associated with sciatica. Transcutaneous electrical nerve stimulation (TENS) blocks pain signals by sending electrical currents into the muscles through electrodes taped to the skin. It is a painless process. Ultrasound uses deep therapeutic heat produced on sound waves for soft tissue healing. And simple cold packs and hot packs provide pain relief, as well.

There are also techniques that work to overcome weakness and to improve flexibility. Proprioceptive neuromuscular facilitation (PNF)—in simple terms, a process of progressively stretching and then relaxing muscles with the assistance of a practitioner—and manipulation increase joint range of motion and strength. Traction, which involves gently drawing and pulling muscles, stretches the spine and is used especially in cases of disc injury. Finally, exercise programs increase the strength of the muscles in the back and abdomen, as well as increase endurance and flexibility. All of the above-discussed physical therapy approaches can be outpatient treatments.

Surgery

Surgery is less common now. Noninvasive therapy is predominantly recommended, because people with sciatica usually recover on their own within six weeks. Yet sometimes surgery is performed. For example, an operation may be conducted to remove a herniated disc or parts of a disc. In the case of massive disc deterioration, surgery may be performed to fuse two or more vertebrae together, thus improving function and strength of the spine.

Other Conventional Treatments

Conventional medicine generally suggests bed rest for a limit of one or two days. Prolonged bed rest is usually discouraged, as it can lead to an increase in low back pain. In addition, pain management groups and stress management groups are often recommended to encourage relaxation of the body and mind.

COMPLEMENTARY MEDICINE'S APPROACH

Complementary medicine connects easily into the present conventional approach for the treatment of low back pain. The complementary approach takes into account the whole person—the holistic philosophy—and also strives to avoid invasive treatments. A key element is the belief that the mind influences the body and the body, in turn, has an impact on the mind. Hence, there is an emphasis on the body's ability to heal itself with the help of natural, noninvasive therapies that are effective and without harmful side effects.

Complementary medicine supports client education, as clients take a very active role in their own healing, and encourages positive lifestyle changes. This can mean making changes that range anywhere from nutrition to the way you get up from a chair or vacuum a carpet. Its approaches are not viewed as *alternatives*, but as *complements* to conventional medicine. In some instances, complementary medicine may arise as the primary treatment. Consider the following trends for the growing use and acceptance of complementary medicine:

- The prevalence of complementary medicine use has increased by 25 percent, from 33.8 percent in 1990 to 42.1 percent in 1997.[4]

- The total number of visits to complementary medicine providers increased by 47 percent, from 427 million in 1990 to 629 million in 1997.[5]

- The total number of visits to complementary medicine providers (629 million) exceeded the total number of visits to all primary care physicians (386 million) in 1997.[6]

- From 1990 to 1997, estimated expenditures for complementary medicine professional services increased by 45 percent, exclusive of inflation, and in 1997 were estimated at $21.2 billion.[7]

- Out-of-pocket expenditures for complementary medicine professional services in 1997 were estimated at $12.2 billion. This exceeded the out-of-pocket expenditures for all U.S. hospitalizations.[8]

- In 1997, total out-of-pocket expenditures relating to complementary therapies were conservatively estimated at $27 billion. This is comparable to the projected out-of-pocket expenditures for all U.S. physician services.[9]

- Sixty-four percent of the U.S. medical schools reported offering courses on complementary and alternative medicine, as indicated in a study published in 1998.[10]

- By 1995, approximately 60 to 90 percent of medical doctors were making referrals to some form of complementary medicine.[11]

- The *Journal of the American Medical Association* editorial board and senior staff, and the editors of the *American Medical Association Archives* journals ranked alternative medicine in the top three subjects (of eighty-six) to cover in 1998.[12]

With facts like these, it is not hard to identify complementary medicine's approach as a significant and promising avenue of treatment in medicine today.

Beginning of Research

With the increasing demand for and acceptance of complementary medicine, the need for randomized and controlled research studies on its effectiveness for particular conditions is evident. This research is presently developing and is receiving national support through the National Center for Complementary and Alternative Medicine (NCCAM), originally established as the Office of Alternative Medicine at the National Institutes of Health in 1992. It was upgraded to a national center in 1998. Ongoing studies using a single complementary approach for a specific condition are in progress. Research centers have also been established to study a variety of approaches for a range of conditions. These findings will help to enhance the validity, accuracy, and acceptance of complementary medicine in the future. For more information on current complementary approach research issues, see page 117.

Along with proof from valid scientific studies, the issue of one's belief in the healing potential of specific therapeutic approaches, conventional and/or complementary, will always have a powerful effect on treatment outcomes. With sciatica and most low back problems, symptoms tend to clear up naturally over a period of time.[13] The question then remains, did the treatments really work or would the condition have gone away on its own? Even with this question, however, treatments may accelerate the process of recovery, make the painful stages more bearable, prevent recurrences, and enable the individual to have a more positive attitude toward recovery, thus aiding the overall healing process.

Selection of Approaches

In Part II, we explain various complementary medicine approaches that may help relieve the discomforts of sciatica. Since scientific research on the efficacy of complementary medicine is in its beginning stages, our focus in choosing healing approaches for sciatica in this book took into account emerging trends in treatment research and, in addition, the underlying causes of sciatica. We considered the following causes when deciding on which complementary medicine approaches to discuss: strained or weak muscles; improper body mechanics and movements; poor posture; and the effects of stress, anxiety, and negative thinking. Our recommended approaches for healing and recovery target one or more of these categories and offer gradual relief from pain.

Please keep in mind that we support an integrative approach for dealing with sciatica, promoting the combined benefits of both conventional and complementary medicine. There are circumstances when a physician will be essential in the diagnosis of a condition, particularly in cases of lumbar herniated discs, spinal stenosis, ruptured discs, arthritis, endometrial cysts, ankylosing spondylitis, and sacroiliac ligament tears. We strongly recommend that the integrated approach be coordinated with the help of a physician.

Our range of complementary treatment options for sciatica addresses both physical and emotional components. For example, using proper body mechanics, correcting posture, and strengthening the supporting muscles of the body not only assist in physical healing and in pain reduction, but have profound effects in stimulating positive emotions. By integrating both the physical and psychological components of the pain cycle, the patient's well-being and recovery is better addressed.

Issues to Consider

There are quite a few things to think about when you are choosing a complementary medicine approach. As you read through Part II of this book and weigh the approaches according to what is most acceptable, convenient, and desirable to you, keep the following questions in mind. They will aid you in making final decisions about your treatment program.

❑ Are you comfortable with the physical aspects of the approach—the amount of physical contact with the practitioner; any devices (such as acupuncture needles) or environments (such as the pool in aquatic therapy) necessary; etc.?

❑ Are you comfortable with the psychological components of the approach? Does it fit well into your belief system? Are you entering into treatment with an open and optimistic mindset?

❑ Have you chosen a practitioner who either comes well-recommended or whom you have thoroughly researched, and whose office is easily accessible from your location?

❑ Have you set up a reasonable time frame in which you would like to see results?

❑ Have you reviewed any applicable parameters involving your health insurance plan? (For information on complementary medicine and health insurance issues, see page 121.)

❑ If you are being treated by a physician or other healthcare professional, have you discussed your treatment selection with him or her? (Please note that not all conventional practitioners will be knowledgeable about complementary medicine treatments. It is helpful to inform your conventional practitioner about the approach you are involved in or are considering, and to provide him or her with any available written information, if appropriate. An open dialogue with your healthcare provider can encourage an integrated treatment plan for your optimal health.)

❑ Does your lifestyle match up well with the commitments necessary for effective treatment? In other words, have you taken into consideration: the commute; the number of times per week/month that you will be attending sessions; the feasibility of at-home techniques; and the likely duration of treatment? (Don't forget to consider the option of home or office sessions, depending on your needs and finances.)

It is important to realize that the purpose of incorporating the approaches of complementary medicine into a treatment program is not to replace conventional treatments for sciatica. Instead, it is to provide choices based on an individual's particular needs and preferences. According to Dr. Robert Shields, an osteopathic physician, "One of the most important things to keep in mind is that pain is caused by a variety of underlying problems, and it is naive to think that one modality will help improve all back pain."[14]

A recent study published in the *Journal of Orthopedic and Sports Physical Therapy* recommends that complementary medicine approaches be part of the standard treatment protocol for low back problems. This report states that the standard protocol should include three components: relaxation approaches for pain; manual techniques and exercises to correct physical alignment; and movement/mobilization techniques to improve posture and movement patterns. The reasons cited for the interest in complementary medicine for the treatment of low back pain are the fact that 80 percent of the patients suffering from low back pain show no pathological cause and from the growing frustration of practitioners and clients with the outcome of traditional treatment protocols.[15] Individuals have a greater chance of returning to an optimal state of health and reducing the risk of recurrence by combining approaches that break the chronic pain cycle; improve postural habits and movement patterns; increase strength, flexibility and endurance; relax the body and mind; and encourage positive changes in lifestyle, diet, and negative thinking patterns.

Conclusion

Relief from the painful symptoms of sciatica often comes with establishing a new way of living. A person's treatment success will depend on his or her willingness to continue learning and trying changes in lifestyle over the course of time. So it is important not to underestimate your own role in your healing process.

The overall goal of the most effective sciatica treatment program is to encourage a positive state of mind using techniques of belief, relaxation, and stress reduction, in conjunction with other therapeutic approaches designed to suit the physical and emotional needs of each person. Some people will need greater work on spinal alignment, muscular healing, and proper posture. Others will find considerable relief from learning stress management. Making efforts to address both the physical and emotional components of the healing process speak to the harmonious way that conventional and complementary medicine can work together in the alleviation of painful sciatica symptoms.

PART II

Treatment Approaches

The interrelatedness of the mind and body is a basic philosophy of complementary medicine—that is, your state of mind can powerfully affect physical symptoms, and physical states have strong effects on emotions. For example, maintaining proper body mechanics, correcting posture, and strengthening the supporting muscles of the body not only assist in physical healing and in pain reduction, but have profound effects in stimulating positive emotions. The positive emotions, in turn, encourage further healing and well-being. Our selected range of complementary treatment options for sciatica, therefore, addresses the physical components of pain, body mechanics, and activity habits, as well as the emotional components of negative thinking, anxiety, and life stressors.

Part II offers detailed explanations of over fifteen approaches. Read through the various options and then choose to further explore the options with which you feel most comfortable. Remember, also, to utilize the expertise of your physician or other healthcare provider in the initial assessment process. As you progress through treatment services, inform you healthcare provider on how the approaches are working to relieve your sciatica. Maintaining open communication between the conventional and complementary components of your treatment will help you to integrate your treatments most effectively. You may need to gather a little courage and motivation to try a new approach, but a lot of comfort and hope are likely to be gained.

ACUPRESSURE

WHAT IS IT?

Acupressure is a simple, noninvasive technique based on the philoso-phies of Traditional Chinese Medicine (TCM). The main concept behind TCM is that healing energy—*chi*—circulates throughout the body along specific pathways called *meridians*. The unobstructed movement of chi throughout the body is necessary for health. The flow of chi along the meridians connects all areas of the body like the streets on a road map link various locations. So it is possible, for example, to treat back pain by applying pressure to a specific section of the knee, because a meridian connects the two areas.

The goal of acupressure, which can be described as an ancient system of massage, is to stimulate, disperse, and regulate the body's healing energy. Through the practitioner's application of pressure, using fingers, palms, thumbs, or elbows, chi is encouraged to circu-late throughout the body.

HOW DOES ACUPRESSURE VIEW THE PROBLEM OF SCIATICA?

According to the philosophies of TCM and, therefore, acupressure, disruption in the even flow of chi to the meridians can create pain and illness anywhere in the body. Sciatica occurs when there is an obstruction in the bladder, gallbladder, or kidney meridians, result-ing in poor circulation of chi and blood along those pathways. These meridians affect the low back. The obstruction is believed to arise when cold, wind, or dampness invade the body and lodge in the meridians. If cold is the cause, the sciatic pain will be more intense.

HOW DOES ACUPRESSURE TREAT SCIATICA?

During an acupressure session, the practitioner takes a full medical history, including examination through observation and questioning. He or she addresses all relevant information, characteristics, and symptoms. The acupressurist will then check the alignment of your spine. Results from this evaluation determine the specific acupressure areas on which the practitioner works.

There are particular locations along the meridians, called acupressure points, where the chi can be guided by applying firm pressure. As a practitioner applies pressure to these points, obstructions in the flow of healing energy dissolves, muscles and ligaments relax, and the body returns to a healthier state. By moving the stagnation and dispersing the wind, cold, or damp, the kidney, gallbladder, and/or bladder meridians are strengthened. As a result, the symptoms of sciatica decrease. Applicable acupressure points could be along the low back and legs, and/or at distal points on other parts of the body. If points are used along the low back and legs, some of these points may be tender and sore while being treated.

A completed acupressure session results in effects that are similar to those achieved by massage, including: increased blood and nutrient circulation; the release of tension in muscle fibers; the release of endorphins, which are brain chemicals that serve as the body's natural opiates or pain killers; and the elimination of waste matter, especially lactic acid, from the muscle. Because acupressure dislodges toxins, you may experience a sensation of lightheadedness, but it will pass quickly. To cleanse the system, it is recommended that you drink plenty of water after a treatment session.

Quick Tip

To prevent injury to your back when sneezing, bend your knees and brace your back by holding onto a nearby support.

IS THERE CURRENT RELEVANT RESEARCH?

There are numerous studies that confirm the beneficial effects of *acupuncture* points for pain relief. (See Acupuncture, page 30.) However, scientific studies on the beneficial effects of *acupressure* points are limited. The field of acupressure is in need of studies that follow standard research protocol in order to validate its effectiveness.

WHAT IS THE ESTIMATED COST AND DURATION
OF TREATMENT?

Generally, an acupressure session costs $40 to $80 and lasts for 60 minutes. As sciatica is a chronic problem, a number of sessions are often necessary before the body experiences a significant result.

IS MY HEALTH INSURANCE LIKELY TO COVER
THIS TREATMENT?

Some health plans cover for acupressure, but the parameters of coverage vary. If your health plan covers some form of complementary medicine, it would be best to contact the person in charge of the complementary medicine portion of the policy and speak to him or her directly regarding the specifics of coverage. Also, it is possible that your health plan covers complementary medicine and you are not aware of it. In either case, contacting your health-plan organization and speaking to a knowledgeable representative would yield the best results.

WHAT CREDENTIALS AND/OR EDUCATIONAL
BACKGROUND SHOULD I LOOK FOR
IN A PRACTITIONER?

There are no state requirements for practicing acupressure in the United States. However, choose a practitioner who has graduated from and has been certified by an accredited school of acupressure. The American Oriental Bodywork Therapy Association, listed on page 30, requires that its members meet certain professional and academic standards. Therefore, getting a referral from this organization will guarantee you that the practitioner has received proper training.

Some acupressure practitioners use *OBT*, indicating Oriental Bodywork Therapist, after their names. Others indicate that they belong to particular professional groups. And while acupressure is an approach unto itself, health professionals in other fields may be trained and effective practitioners of acupressure.

WHAT PROFESSIONAL ORGANIZATION CAN I CONTACT FOR FURTHER INFORMATION?

American Oriental Bodywork Therapy Association
Laurel Oak Corporate Center, Suite 408
1010 Haddenfield-Berlin Road
Voorhees, NJ 08043
Phone: (609) 782–1616

ACUPUNCTURE

WHAT IS IT?

Acupuncture is an ancient Chinese method of healing that is based on the philosophies of Traditional Chinese Medicine (TCM). These philosophies hold that universal life energy—*chi*—is present in every living creature and circulates throughout the body along specific pathways called *meridians.* Unobstructed flow of chi along the meridians is necessary for well-being. The meridians connect various parts of the body to each other. So it is possible, for example, to treat back pain by treating points on a particular area of the knee, thereby stimulating the movement of chi along a particular pathway and initiating a healing process.

Acupuncture involves the insertion of fine needles at specific points on the meridians. The penetration of these points triggers the flow of chi, resolves blockages, and allows recovery to begin. The primary focus of acupuncture is to correct the cause of illness by stimulating the body's natural healing abilities.

HOW DOES ACUPUNCTURE VIEW THE PROBLEM OF SCIATICA?

The philosophy behind TCM and, therefore, acupuncture is that disruption in the even flow of chi throughout the meridians can create pain and illness anywhere in the body. Sciatica occurs when there is an obstruction in the bladder, gallbladder, or kidney meridians, resulting in poor circulation of chi and blood along those pathways.

These meridians affect the low back. The obstruction is believed to arise when cold, wind, or dampness lodge in the meridians. If cold is the cause, the sciatic pain will be more intense.

HOW DOES ACUPUNCTURE TREAT SCIATICA?

During an acupuncture session, the practitioner takes a full medical history, including examination through observation and questioning. He or she addresses all relevant information, characteristics, and symptoms. Results from this evaluation determine the cause of the problem and which specific acupuncture points will be treated.

The acupuncturist stimulates the circulation of chi by inserting needles into points in specific muscles, relieving the blockages that are causing back pain. By restoring the circulation of chi and increasing blood flow to these areas, muscle spasms are decreased and weak muscles are strengthened. For variations on the needle-insertion technique, see "Additional Acupuncture Techniques" on page 32.

Treatments are practically, if not completely, painless. The needles are sterile, disposable, hair-thin, and generally cause no bleeding. You may feel a slight tingling, or a small amount of heat or numbness, as the needle reaches the acupuncture point. However, these sensations are fleeting. Often, the individual is completely unaware that the needle is being inserted.

According to conventional medicine's analysis of acupuncture, the stimulation of acupuncture points rouses the body's natural healing abilities to regulate red and white blood cell counts. It also triggers the production of endorphins and enkephalins (natural pain killers), as well as cortisol (an anti-inflammatory agent). In addition, the stimulation promotes healthier blood pressure. Treating particular acupuncture points can even help relieve depression and anxiety, which are symptoms that can accompany low back pain.

One of the greatest advantages of this approach is the absence of any harmful side effects associated with its use. Patients sometimes report feeling lightheaded, even euphoric, after treatments. In order to stabilize the body, a few moments of rest after a session is advised, in addition to drinking fluids to flush out toxins that have been released by the treatment.

Additional Acupuncture Techniques

There are several acupuncture treatments that differ from or are variations of the widely known technique of needle insertion. Four methods that are effective for sciatica are described below.

Cupping—Specialized glass cups are placed upon specific acupuncture points on the kidney meridian, located on the low back. A process of removing the oxygen from the cup creates a vacuum-like pressure. This pressure draws chi and blood to the area of the lower back, facilitating the flow of chi and opening the meridians.

Electro-acupuncture—After acupuncture needles have been inserted, a low-intensity, pulsing, electric current is applied through the acupuncture needle. Electro-acupuncture disperses a tingling sensation around the acupuncture point and reaches a large number of acupuncture points on the meridian. It is particularly effective for the relief of pain.

Laser acupuncture—Laser acupuncture is an option for individuals who fear needles. Acupuncture points are stimulated by a fine, low-energy laser beam emitted from a laser pen. The treatment is painless.

Moxibustion—Moxibustion is a form of heat therapy. It involves the burning of a cigar-shaped roll of the herb moxa—also known as mugwort, or Artemisia vulgaris—above the acupuncture point. An additional technique includes laying a small slice of fresh gingerroot directly on the treatment site, and then placing a piece of dried moxa on top of the ginger. The moxa is ignited, quickly burns on the ginger slice, and the juice from the ginger permeates the aching area.

Moxibustion results in a deep, penetrating heat and subsequent pain relief. The heat not only has a soothing effect, but also opens the pores of the skin, allowing the healing properties of the ginger to penetrate the body. Ginger is known for its ability to provide internal warmth. Moxibustion is an extremely effective treatment for conditions of weakness and sensitivity to cold.

IS THERE CURRENT RELEVANT RESEARCH?

There have been many studies done to assess the effectiveness of acupuncture for back problems. The National Institutes of Health recently convened a twelve-person consensus panel of impartial experts in the medical field. After reviewing hundreds of studies in the field of acupuncture, their results stated clearly that the data supporting the efficacy of acupuncture for a variety of conditions, including low back pain, was strong. The panel concluded that acupuncture for low back pain was useful as an adjunct treatment, an acceptable alternative, or as part of a comprehensive treatment program.[1]

WHAT IS THE ESTIMATED COST AND DURATION OF TREATMENT?

Generally, an acupuncture session costs $40 to $80 and lasts for approximately 50 minutes. Because sciatica tends to be a chronic problem, repeated sessions are often necessary for long-term relief. For chronic conditions, a series of six to ten treatment sessions is typical. Having sessions in close proximity to each other—for example, having two or three sessions in 1 week—yields a more effective result.

IS MY HEALTH INSURANCE LIKELY TO COVER THIS TREATMENT?

Many health plans cover for acupuncture, but the parameters of coverage vary. If your health plan covers some form of complementary medicine, it would be best to contact the person in charge of the complementary medicine portion of the policy and speak to him or her directly regarding the specifics of coverage. Also, it is possible that your health plan covers complementary medicine and you are not aware of it. In either case, contacting your health-plan organization and speaking to a knowledgeable representative would yield the best results.

WHAT CREDENTIALS AND/OR EDUCATIONAL BACKGROUND SHOULD I LOOK FOR IN A PRACTITIONER?

Requirements for the practice of acupuncture differ from state to state. Some states do not require practitioners to graduate from accredited programs, but a growing number of states have instituted this as a prerequisite for state licensure. If you are selecting a nonphysician acupuncturist, be sure to choose one who has more than two years of training at an accredited program, is licensed or registered in your state if applicable, and/or has passed the National Commission for the Certification of Acupuncturists (NCCA) exam, which requires more than 1,000 hours of acupuncture training. Safe standards have been established by the NCCA. Practitioners who are certified by the NCCA or by the state follow strict regulations for the proper sterilization of equipment, the use of disposable needles, and proper needle handling.

Some medical doctors practice acupuncture. If you decide to follow this route, choose a physician who has had at least 200 hours of acupuncture training and has earned membership in the American Academy of Medical Acupuncture, which requires proof of training.

The following are credential initials that apply to acupuncturists: *CA*, Certified Acupuncturist; *DiplAc*, Diplomat in Acupuncture; *LAc/LicAc*, Licensed Acupuncturist; *MAc*, Master of Acupuncture; and *RAc*, Registered Acupuncturist.

WHAT PROFESSIONAL ORGANIZATION CAN I CONTACT FOR FURTHER INFORMATION?

National Acupuncture and Oriental Medicine Alliance
14637 Starr Road, SE
Olalla, WA 98359
(253) 851–6896

THE ALEXANDER TECHNIQUE

WHAT IS IT?

Observe the posture of children—the way they hold their heads and backs. Compare it with the parents' posture. The difference is startling. The children move with ease and lightness, while the parents are not as fluid in their movements and their posture is not as connected. The Alexander Technique helps adults to eliminate long-established poor postural habits. Through this treatment, individuals relearn how to move their bodies with greater ease, much like they once did as children. The main objective is to develop conscious control of your movements in all activities through achievable goals.

The Alexander Technique is mostly taught in one-on-one sessions, where the practitioner is referred to as a teacher and the client is recognized as a student. The lesson focuses on movement, and may center on something as basic as getting up from a chair. The instructor directs the student carefully, according to his or her particular needs. This self-care program allows a person to make positive, conscious changes to posture and movement habits. The goal, over time, is for these new patterns to become second nature.

HOW DOES THE ALEXANDER TECHNIQUE VIEW THE PROBLEM OF SCIATICA?

The majority of back problems, including sciatica, are direct results of not using the supporting muscles of the body properly. Poor postural habits and unhealthy body mechanics, such as slouching in a chair or lifting objects without bending the knees, can lead to aches, pains, muscle tightness, and the inability to function properly. In addition, the human head, which can account for up to 15 percent of the body's total weight, is supported by the spinal column. The weight tends to pull the head forward, forcing support muscles of the neck to keep it balanced. Any abnormal posture can put unnecessary stress and burden on the spinal column, not allowing it to carry the head properly. Back problems occur as a result.

Unnecessary tension on the back's supporting muscles is the major cause of back pain. Tense muscles lose their flexibility, becoming not only painful but more susceptible to injury. As a result of muscle stiffness and injury, inflammation and misalignments in structure may occur. And these problems can lead to compression of the sciatic nerve—sciatica. The Alexander Technique emphasizes that the entire spine and back must be used correctly in order to stop pain in any particular area of the back.

HOW DOES THE ALEXANDER TECHNIQUE TREAT THE PROBLEM OF SCIATICA?

Before beginning instruction, the teacher conducts an examination through observation and questioning. He or she observes your posture and body mechanics during various activities, as well as any areas of muscular tension. Then the practitioner focuses on specific movements.

The Alexander Technique works towards correcting bad habits. The instructor teaches simple exercises designed to improve balance, posture, and coordination. He or she also offers gentle hands-on guidance and verbal instruction to train you in the optimal use of your body. You will learn to maintain a more relaxed posture and more controlled movement patterns that will balance the body and relax neck muscles. The Alexander Technique aims to free the neck from taking an active, primary role for all movements of the body.

Quick Tip

The pressure on your spine from sitting can be quite intense. When selecting a chair for your office or your home computer, choose a chair with no arms. Adjust the seat height so that when your low back is pressed against the back of the chair, your feet are flat on the floor and your knees are a little higher than your hips.

Benefits of this approach include a release of excess tension in the body and a lengthening of the spine to eliminate compression. You will experience greater freedom and flexibility in movement, as well as improved posture, appearance, and general health. Upon completion of training, you should be able to correct yourself immediately when destructive habits return.

IS THERE CURRENT RELEVANT RESEARCH?

In a study conducted through Tel Aviv University, Israel, in 1996, a group of sixty-seven chronic back-pain sufferers responded positively to a multidisciplinary treatment approach that included the Alexander Technique as one of the primary treatments. Also included in the comprehensive program were acupuncture, chiropractic, and psychological intervention. The study was 4 weeks in duration. The participants were tested at the 4-week mark and, again, at 6 months. Improvements were maintained throughout the entire time.

The study also demonstrated that results were affected by a person's psychological disposition.[1]

In a 1988 study conducted through the Royal National Orthopaedic Hospital, England, thirty-four chronic pain sufferers whose most common diagnosis was "back pain with radiation to one or both legs" benefited from a comprehensive, behavioral pain-management program that included the Alexander Technique. Results showed improvements in disability ratings and increases in activity levels. The Alexander Technique was rated as the most effective approach used in the pain program.[2]

WHAT IS THE COST AND DURATION OF TREAMENT?

Generally, an Alexander Technique session costs $50 to $85 and lasts for approximately 30 to 50 minutes. The number of sessions necessary for effective changes depends on the severity of your sciatica and on your motivation. However, for most conditions, the average number of Alexander Technique sessions is thirty. How often the sessions occur within a given time period varies considerably.

IS MY HEALTH INSURANCE LIKELY TO COVER
THIS TREATMENT?

Some health plans cover for the Alexander Technique, but the parameters of coverage vary. If your health plan covers some form of complementary medicine, it would be best to contact the person in charge of the complementary medicine portion of the policy and speak to him or her directly regarding the specifics of coverage. Also, it is possible that your health plan covers complementary medicine and you are not aware of it. In either case, contacting your health-plan organization and speaking to a knowledgeable representative would yield the best results.

WHAT CREDENTIALS AND/OR EDUCATIONAL
BACKGROUND SHOULD I LOOK FOR IN A PRACTITIONER?

An instructor of the Alexander Technique must be certified by the North American Society of Teachers of the Alexander Technique (NASTAT). Look for the *NASTAT* initials after the practitioner's name. This credential indicates that the instructor has completed a 3-year, 1,600-hour training program at an approved school.

WHAT PROFESSIONAL ORGANIZATION CAN I CONTACT FOR FURTHER INFORMATION?

North American Society of Teachers of the Alexander Technique
3010 Hennepin Avenue S, Suite 10
Minneapolis, MN 55408
(800) 473–0620

IS THERE A HELPFUL AT-HOME TECHNIQUE THAT I CAN USE?

To help prevent or reduce a muscle spasm in your back, get on your hands and knees and slowly crawl forward six to eight steps, then backward six to eight steps. This easy motion helps to relax tight muscles.

AQUATIC THERAPY

WHAT IS IT?

Aquatic therapy, also known as water therapy, has been used for centuries to invigorate the body and relieve pain. The exercises, which consist of stretching and relaxation techniques, take place in a warm, shallow pool that is specifically designed for therapeutic purposes. Many aquatic therapy facilities are equipped with a heated pool (92° F to 99° F), as well as an additional pool containing cooler water. Aquatic therapy is particularly useful for treating muscle and joint pain, as well as for relieving stress.

HOW DOES AQUATIC THERAPY VIEW THE PROBLEM OF SCIATICA?

No matter what the cause of low back pain, water therapy has been considered the perfect medium for relaxing muscles and accelerating the healing process. Whether the sciatic nerve is irritated by a protruding disc, bone spurs, inflamed tissue around the spinal joint, muscle spasm, athletic injury, or tight muscles as a result of excess stress, the buoyancy of water is therapeutic to the body and soothing to the mind.

HOW DOES AQUATIC THERAPY TREAT SCIATICA?

The warm water used for aquatic therapy stimulates and then relaxes tired, aching muscles. It increases blood flow to the skin and muscles, thus relieving stiffness. By improving the circulation, a fresh supply of oxygen and nutrients are carried to the tissue to repair damage. The cooler, more invigorating water helps reduce muscle swelling and pain by constricting the blood vessels.

Quick Tip

Ice reduces swelling and can also help to alleviate the pain from back-muscle strain. Applied to the painful area, ice will numb sore tissue. Fill a paper cup with water and allow it to freeze in your freezer. Peel the paper back and you will be ready for an ice massage. Move the ice continuously over the site of your pain for 4 to 5 minutes. Once the swelling has decreased, the application of heat may provide further relief.

Gentle and rhythmic movements are performed from seated, standing, walking, and/or floating positions. In addition to targeting problem areas particular to the lower back, the stretching and conditioning activities are designed to benefit all major muscle groups, decrease muscle stiffness, and calm the mind. The goal of aquatic therapy is to develop freer body movements that increase strength, flexibility, and endurance. You will begin with guidance from the instructor and gradually learn to manage your own therapy program. With a decrease in tension, improvements in your musculature, and, therefore, improvements in spinal alignment, the sciatic nerve is less likely to be compressed or obstructed.

IS THERE CURRENT RELEVANT RESEARCH?

To our knowledge, there are no published scientific studies on the effectiveness of aquatic therapy specifically for the relief of sciatica. However, studies do indicate that aquatic therapy can improve over-all fitness levels of participants and has been used successfully in back rehabilitation programs to increase muscular and cardiovascular endurance.[1]

For example, in 1983, Vickery, Cureton, and Langstaff studied the physiological benefits of a water aerobics program that involved the activities of aquatic calisthenics, jogging in place, and modified lap-swimming. They demonstrated that heart rate and oxygen uptake significantly increased among the participants.[2] Thus, the study subjects were receiving the benefits of intense exercise in a comfortable, low-impact environment.

Heberlein, Perez, Wygand, and Commons, in a 1989 unpublished study at Adelphi University in New York, concluded that water aerobics significantly changed body composition and improved fitness. They compared the effects of land versus water aerobics and found that the water exercisers used a greater percentage of fat as a fuel source during 30-minute exercise periods.[3]

WHAT IS THE ESTIMATED COST AND DURATION OF TREATMENT?

Generally, an aquatic therapy class costs about $20 and lasts for approximately 30 to 60 minutes. In order to achieve significant results, commit to a series of at least six to eight sessions.

IS MY HEALTH INSURANCE LIKELY TO COVER THIS TREATMENT?

Most health plans cover for aquatic therapy, but coverage is usually for a specific number of sessions. Therefore, it is beneficial for you to learn the techniques in order to continue the aquatic exercises on your own at a local "Y," at a health club, or in your own pool. In doing so, you can greatly enhance the recovery process and decrease the possibility of re-injury by maintaining a regular, therapeutic exercise program.

Hydrotherapy

Hydrotherapy is the application of water in its various forms (liquid, solid, and vapor) for purposes of health treatment. Often a practitioner will apply alternate hot and cold compresses to the painful area of the back. The various applications of hot and cold water treatments create different physiological effects in the body. These effects can be either stimulating or sedating to the nervous and circulatory systems. For example, short applications of cold can have a stimulating effect, while longer applications of cold can have a sedating effect.

Hydrotherapy offers many different treatment options, some of which are:

- *hot/cold packs*
- *Jacuzzi*
- *sitz bath*

- *hot tubs*
- *moist heat packs*
- *steam baths*

- *ice massage*
- *saunas*
- *whirlpool*

Both hydrotherapy and aquatic therapy rely on the natural healing effects of water. Hydrotherapy differs from aquatic therapy in that the client passively receives the water-based treatment; unlike aquatic therapy, there is no exercise routine involved.

WHAT CREDENTIALS AND/OR EDUCATIONAL BACKGROUND SHOULD I LOOK FOR IN A PRACTITIONER?

There are no mandatory requirements or state regulations for aquatic therapists. However, we recommend that you select a practitioner who has been certified: he or she should be listed as *Certified Aquatic Exercise Instructor.* Other credentials to look for are CPR and first aid certification, and *WSI,* which signifies Red Cross certification for a trained Water Safety Instructor.

Levels of certification vary; certain facilities look for particular levels. For example, hospital-based programs generally have higher credential requirements than local gyms. Many physical therapy and occupational therapy facilities offer aquatic therapy, as do many health and fitness centers, YMCAs, and YWCAs. Inquire about the training of the practitioners.

WHAT PROFESSIONAL ORGANIZATION CAN I CONTACT FOR FURTHER INFORMATION?

Aquatic Exercise Association
P.O. Box 1609
Nokomis, FL 34274–1609
(941) 486–8600

Red Cross (local chapters found in your Yellow Pages)

CHIROPRACTIC

WHAT IS IT?

The chiropractic system is based on the belief that a strong, agile, and aligned spine is the key to good health. The nervous system of the human body is protected by the spine, and when the spine is in its proper position, the nervous system is free to send out the necessary signals for the body to function normally. When there is misalignment to the vertebrae of the spine, disharmony anywhere in the body may result, including low back pain.

A doctor of chiropractic medicine uses manipulation of the spine in order to reestablish the proper alignment of the spinal bones and to restore normal motion. Manipulations are performed by hand, although some chiropractic doctors may use special treatment tables to facilitate the outcome. Certain treatment processes also include the application of heat, cold, or ultrasound for muscle relaxation. In addition, a chiropractic session might include dietary advice and nutritional counseling, rehabilitative exercises, and advice on job-related body mechanics.

HOW DOES CHIROPRACTIC MEDICINE VIEW THE PROBLEM OF SCIATICA?

According to chiropractic philosophy, pain is an alarm the body sends off to notify you that something is wrong. To simply tune the alarm out (through pain medication) does not make the physical problem go away. Often, when the symptom of pain is suppressed without finding the cause, a more severe condition or even permanent damage can occur. So first and foremost, your discomfort must be treated.

Chiropractors believe the alignment of the spine is essential for the optimal functioning of the nervous system. As described in Part I of this book, the human spine consists of twenty-four bones called vertebrae. Discs of cartilage between each pair of vertebrae provide protective cushioning. The spinal cord, which is part of the central nervous system, suspends from the brain and runs through the hollow tunnel of the spine. Small nerve trunks branch off the spinal cord and lead through channels in the vertebrae. When the notches in the vertebra are aligned correctly, nerves can pass through and function properly. But if the notches are misaligned, the channel distorts and the nerves become entrapped, compressed, or pinched. Trauma and poor posture are two common factors that can result in unhealthy pressure being applied to the spine. The symptoms of sciatica can develop in such circumstances.

HOW DOES CHIROPRACTIC TREAT SCIATICA?

Through observation, palpation of vertebrae, manual movements (to determine range of motion), and a nerve reflex test, the chiropractor can identify misalignments and muscle weaknesses. The chiropractor's objective is to correct the misalignments through spinal manipulation or adjustments. Special consideration is placed upon the spine's structure and function, including the unobstructed pathways of nerves.

Adjustments to the spine are made by using quick, precise thrusts to move the joints just beyond their normal range of motion. A low force method can also be used, called the Activator Technique. With this technique, the chiropractor manually uses a hand-held instrument to make gentle, precise adjustments. Manual spinal traction, a method of gently pulling and stretching the spinal area, is also used to stretch the vertebrae of the lower back. These forms of manipulation can improve mobility, subsequently decreasing inflammation, pain, nerve irritation, and tightness in the supporting muscles of the back. Additionally, since the back muscles are attached to the spine and give support to the structure, the chiropractor may also integrate

muscle work that uses various massage therapy techniques to alleviate tension and / or spasm.

IS THERE CURRENT RELEVANT RESEARCH?

Scientific research indicates that chiropractic may be the most effective treatment for acute low back pain.[1] In 1992, a review of studies
on the efficacy of chiropractic manipulation for back pain concluded
that chiropractic appears to be an effective treatment, but that more
studies, with improved research methods, are needed in the future.[2]
Then, in 1994, the Agency for Health Care Policy and Research
(AHCPR) concluded that spinal manipulation is effective for acute
low back pain. They recommended spinal manipulation instead of
prescription drugs, surgery, or other expensive, technical procedures.[3]

In 1996, another study that reviewed the literature on chiropractic concluded that the efficacy of spinal manipulation for patients
with acute or chronic low back pain had not been demonstrated with
sound, randomized clinical trials. However, researchers recognized
that there are indications that manipulation might be effective in
some groups of patients with low back pain.[4] This was followed by
additional research. In 1998, Ian Coulter, PhD, published a review
article in *Integrative Medicine* on the efficacy and risks of chiropractic
manipulation. He included a major study conducted by the Rand
Corporation, which confirmed the effectiveness of chiropractic
manipulation for the treatment of acute low back pain.[5]

On a smaller scale, also in 1998, a study followed one patient with
sciatica and a herniated disc. She suffered from low back and leg pain
that was increasing in severity over a 6-day period. Nine chiropractic
treatments were required before she was released from care with improved symptoms. The study, although extremely limited, concluded
that the nonsurgical, conservative approach of chiropractic care should
be completed for disc herniations before considering surgery.[6]

WHAT IS THE ESTIMATED COST AND DURATION
OF TREATMENT?

Generally, the initial chiropractic visit costs $50 to $100, depending on diagnostic testing and the individual practitioner's rates, and lasts for approximately 30 to 60 minutes. Many chiropractors offer free consultations. Follow-up visits usually cost $20 to $50 and last about 10 to 20 minutes. Treatment should be effective within two to fifteen visits, depending on the severity of your sciatica.

IS MY HEALTH INSURANCE LIKELY TO COVER THIS TREATMENT?

Some form of coverage for chiropractic care is available in all fifty states, but the parameters of coverage vary. Contact your health-plan organization and speak to a knowledgeable representative regarding the specifics of coverage.

Quick Tip

When sitting in a chair to read, avoid slumping over and bringing your face to the book. Instead, sit with your feet flat on the floor, slide all the way to the back of the seat, and, if helpful, use a small pillow behind the low-back area for added support. Place another pillow on your lap to raise the level of the book for easier reading. Finally, rest your feet on a book or low-level footstool, thus allowing your knees to be slightly higher than your hips. This is the best position.

WHAT CREDENTIALS AND/OR EDUCATIONAL BACKGROUND SHOULD I LOOK FOR IN A PRACTITIONER?

A chiropractor must have the initials *DC*, which indicates Doctor of Chiropractic, after his or her name. All states require chiropractic doctors to be licensed. This means that they must graduate from an accredited college of chiropractic to earn the DC degree, then pass an examination from the National Board of Chiropractic Examiners, and pass a state board exam. In order to keep their licenses, chiropractors are required to fulfill continuing education hours each year.

WHAT PROFESSIONAL ORGANIZATION CAN I CONTACT FOR FURTHER INFORMATION?

American Chiropractic Association
1701 Clarendon Boulevard
Arlington, VA 22209
(800) 986–4636

EMOTIONAL PAIN RELIEF THERAPY

WHAT IS IT?

Emotions play a vital role in our lives. When they are bottled up inside, the internal pressure can lead to an increase in anxiety, anger, depression, guilt, dysfunctional behavior, and even physical pain. So it is a reality that, as the mind struggles with life events and emotional reactions to them, the body can manifest the struggle in physical pain, often occurring in the back, neck, shoulder, and buttocks regions. Stress, pent-up emotions, and/or repressed emotions directly affect the way our bodies feel. Repressed emotions refer to feelings that are not directly accessible to the conscious mind; in order to work through them, they have to be explored along with related experiences and feelings, usually under the guidance of a psychotherapist.

Emotional pain relief therapy refers to a form of psychotherapy during which the focus is on the internal issues and feelings that are affecting the body's pain. Psychotherapy is a process of talking—a discussion between a trained psychotherapist and a person struggling with a life problem. It focuses on the healing of the mind and the emotions. The therapeutic methods used to process feelings will vary. However, the goals for emotional pain relief therapy remain constant: an acknowledgment and acceptance that physical pain can be related to emotional issues, a commitment to process these emotions, and a willingness to consciously change the way your mind is responding to everyday stress and life events.

HOW DOES EMOTIONAL PAIN RELIEF THERAPY VIEW THE PROBLEM OF SCIATICA?

Stress often occurs when the continuous demands of life overwhelm our ability to cope with them. These demands (stressors) can be internal, involving emotions and attitudes. They can also be external, involving events that we cannot control, such as traffic and work deadlines. The body reacts to stressors by releasing stress hormones that increase heart rate and breathing rate, as well as tighten muscles throughout the body. Muscular tension can put unhealthy pressure on the spine and, therefore, cause misalignments and obstructed nerve pathways.

Sciatica can be attributed to an irritated or compressed sciatic nerve, possibly occurring when muscles in the area of the nerve tighten. Emotional stress can be either a direct cause or a contributing factor to low back pain, including sciatica. Measures should be taken to bring relaxation to the muscles. Mental approaches such as meditation and psychotherapeutic interventions can help.

John E. Sarno, MD, a physician and professor of rehabilitation medicine, postulates from his work with hundreds of patients that most back, neck, shoulder, and buttock problems are not mechanical dysfunctions, but are emotion-based, resulting from personality and life experiences. He feels that repressed emotions are particularly to blame; due to the body's struggle to deal with repressed emotions, the central nervous system is activated to induce a slight oxygen deprivation to certain muscles, nerves, tendons, and ligaments. This lack of oxygen is the direct cause of the pain, which he calls the Tension Myositis Syndrome, or TMS. People diagnosed with TMS, of which sciatica can be included as a symptom, have experienced enormous success with Sarno's treatment program for pain relief. It includes knowledge of the mind-body pain syndrome and a willingness to approach pain from an emotional perspective. See "Dr. Sarno's Program for Healing Your Back Pain" on page 51 for more information.

HOW DOES EMOTIONAL PAIN RELIEF THERAPY TREAT SCIATICA?

Your reaction to stress and the resulting pent-up or repressed emotions are learned responses that can have physical consequences. You might be acutely aware of your internal and external responses (conscious responses), or you may be unaware of them (unconscious responses). Whether or not you understand the mechanisms of your response, you are acutely aware of being in pain. With the acknowledgment that emotions can affect your pain, a commitment to process these emotions, and a willingness to understand how the mind can bring on physical symptoms, your body will have the opportunity to reverse many of the physical effects brought on by undue stress and emotional backlog. With the added help of relaxation/meditation techniques (see pages 93 to 101), muscle tension and spinal pressure can be reduced, leading to an alleviation of low back pain, including sciatica.

Psychotherapy provides an attentive listener and comfortable, safe surroundings, giving you an opportunity to identify conflicts, to release emotions, and to find useful coping strategies. The sessions, occurring in group settings or individually, can be open-ended exchanges or they can be clearly focused on specific, instructional topics. The treatment methods for emotional pain relief therapy are numerous. All of them can help you to process emotions and learn to better cope with stress. Several techniques are: bioenergetics; cognitive restructuring; core energetics; Gestalt therapy; guided imagery/ visualization; neurolinguistic programming; and stress management.

At the foundation of *bioenergetics* is the view that problems of the mind will physically manifest themselves in the body. If you are anxious, the body will demonstrate this emotion with increased pulse and muscle rigidity. And if your body is functioning well, your mental state will improve. Bioenergetic therapists are trained to read body language and can determine the location of physical tension resulting from repressed feelings. Once this area has been located, psychotherapy, physical exercises, breathing techniques, and various forms of massage can be used to release the muscle tension, increase energy flow in the body, and allow for the processing of emotions. Bioenergetics is often conducted in a group setting.

Cognitive restructuring follows the theory that negative thoughts can trap you in destructive behavior patterns, negative emotions, and uncomfortable physical symptoms. For example, a student who fails a test may say, "I will never get a good report card." This thought process is a set-up for continued feelings of inadequacy. The therapist helps this student by consistently challenging the distorted thoughts with positive, motivating, and realistic thoughts. The practitioner may reply, "Try this way of thinking: I can study better next time and be better prepared. I will have a chance to improve my grades." Cognitive restructuring results in healthier self-esteem, improved behavior, and a reduction of physical symptoms.

Core energetics branches off of bioenergetics. It includes the element of spirituality and suggests that life energy (feelings of pleasure, joy, and love) emanates from an inner core. When this energy is blocked by emotional conflict, dysfunction occurs. Using psychotherapy, bodywork, and spiritual guidance, this technique aims to penetrate the wall of negative emotions so that the vital energy of the core can flow freely. As a result, you are capable of being a more loving, creative, and vibrant person. Core energetics is often conducted in a group setting.

Gestalt therapy concentrates on helping you become more aware of your present feelings and behavior, so that you can achieve a healthy wholeness. "Gestalt," in German, means "whole." This technique uses drama to express feelings. For example, you might be asked to act out the emotions related to a particular situation by using several chairs. One chair would be your shame, another would be your anger, and yet another would be your sadness. You would move from chair to chair, acting out these emotions. This dramatic exercise allows you to recognize and accept each emotional element as part of your whole being. Gestalt techniques are often conducted in group settings and offered at weekend workshops, so that results can be achieved in a concentrated period of time, rather than over many dispersed sessions.

Through *guided imagery/visualization*, you and your therapist work to find mental pictures that will stimulate natural healing responses. You may use your own imagery or work with visualizations suggested by the therapist. The images/visualizations help to alleviate anxiety and to bring about changes in attitude and behavior. They encourage you to work through emotions connected with trauma, illness, or other life circumstances. For example, a woman experiencing stage fright may imagine her fear as a rock. She pictures holding this rock in her hand and turning it into sand, crumbling through her fingers and disappearing. Anytime she performs in front of an audience, the woman can use this visualization to reduce anxiety and increase confidence. Therapists will often teach visualization exercises as self-help tools that you can use outside of therapy.

Neurolinguistic programming (NLP) is a technique designed to reprogram negative patterns. *Neuro* refers to information that is received through the senses and from which patterns of behavior are formed. *Linguistic* pertains to the verbal and non-verbal languages, such as speech patterns and body language, that are used as tools of communication. *Programming* is a term for the set ways in which we organize our experience, behaviors, and thoughts. During a counseling session, the practitioner observes your language, posture, gestures, and physiological changes (such as skin color, eye movements, and breathing). Then he or she works with you to change unconscious patterns of behavior that are negatively effecting your emotional and physical condition. Sometimes, the session includes a technique called *Using Anchors*, which may involve touch. The practitioner anchors you to a positive image by giving you a cue of touch. It is the use of visualization in combination with physical cues—anchors—that reinforce positive beliefs and behaviors. Visual and auditory anchors may also be used, depending on your needs. NLP achieves significant results in a short period of time and provides an empowering self-help tool.

Stress management therapy helps you to cope more effectively with stress, so that the negative effects on the body, mind, and emotions can be reduced. Stress management training combines education on the sources and effects of stress, discussion of your particular stress reactions, and instruction in helpful coping skills. Training can take place in individual or group sessions.

IS THERE CURRENT RELEVANT RESEARCH?

The mind-body connection to physical illness and pain has been researched extensively in well-respected studies over many years. According to Benson and Stuart in *The Wellness Book,* research over the past several decades has resulted in two clear conclusions. The first is that "specific behaviors contribute to illness." For example, habits that involve overindulgence in food, alcohol, tobacco, exercise, narcotics, etc, have severe effects on the body when it comes to developing and recovering from disease. Furthermore, systematic, formal

Dr. Sarno's Program for Healing Your Back Pain

Dr. Sarno's program for eliminating back pain emphasizes knowledge through short-term education on the mind-body pain process and specifically on the Tension Myositis Syndrome (TMS). TMS is the experience of pain resulting from emotional situations and manifesting in different regions of the body. His program encourages the willingness to act on that knowledge by "talking to your brain" with affirmations that will change the messages sent out from your brain.

According to Dr. Sarno, if his program of acquired knowledge and daily affirmations is followed, the pain can disappear permanently. He believes that many physical interventions, such as physical therapy and medication, offer temporary relief, but clients in his program have shown long-term pain recovery, particularly in the neck, shoulder, back, and buttocks regions.

Dr. Sarno states that it is necessary to cease all physical treatment interventions while undergoing his program, in order to reinforce the pain as emotion-based. He also instructs that before any treatment program begins, a person should receive an appropriate medical diagnosis of TMS to screen out clear physical conditions or diseases that would not benefit from his program of pain recovery. Dr. Sarno does not feel it is necessary to specifically work through repressed emotions for the program to be successful. It is through the acknowledgment and acceptance of the mind-body process that the pain cycle is thwarted and through which most of his clients have found relief. He does indicate, however, that some people may need further help through professional psychotherapy to process unconscious emotions and other life matters.[1,2]

treatment approaches—involving organized programs that guide our behavior—can be more helpful in our recovery process than approaches that are randomly performed and not systematically used.

The second conclusion of the research on the mind-body connection is that "psychological and emotional reactions directly affect physiological function." Our physiological states are partly determined by the way we respond—psychologically and emotionally— to our surroundings. The term *psychophysiological interactions* defines this connection. When we are happy and calm, our bodies tend to be functional and relaxed. When we get angry or frightened, we become "emotionally aroused," tense, and our physical reactions become more severe. It has been proven that repeated, long-term physiological reactions that occur in response to stress can contribute to disease and disorders. Because of this intense connection between body and mind, we must resolve the things that cause our bodies to react in unhealthy ways. This includes destructive thoughts, emotions, worries, and burdens. So research clearly supports that effectively dealing with stress and negative, pent-up emotions can have a healthy impact on certain illnesses and the experience of pain.[3]

WHAT IS THE ESTIMATED COST AND DURATION OF TREATMENT?

A general, estimated cost for an individual psychotherapy session is $40 to $150. The session can last anywhere from 30 to 90 minutes. Group therapy costs approximately $15 to $35 per session, and runs for 60 to 120 minutes. However, there is great variation. Cost depends on the training of the practitioner, the location, and your health insurance. Also, the number of appointments, the frequency, and the duration of therapy will vary according to your specific situation.

IS MY HEALTH INSURANCE LIKELY TO COVER THIS TREATMENT?

Psychotherapy completed under the guidance of a licensed psychotherapist, social worker, psychologist, or psychiatrist is covered under most health plans. However, the specific parameters vary. Speak with your health-plan representative for the coverage and restrictions that apply to your individual case.

WHAT CREDENTIALS AND/OR EDUCATIONAL BACKGROUND SHOULD I LOOK FOR IN A PRACTITIONER?

Certification and licensing of psychotherapists vary from state to state, but are generally based on academic degrees, experience, and the passing of an examination. You have several options when it comes to choosing a practitioner. We recommend that you seek a licensed, certified, and/or qualified psychotherapist in one of the disciplines described below. Please note that some practitioners list only their certification and/or licensing, not their full training. Therefore, it is best to inquire about the full training of a recommended practitioner. He or she may have more experience than is evident from the listing or business card.

Social workers can serve as trained psychotherapists. Applicable degrees and credentials include: *BCD*, Board Certified Diplomate in Clinical Social Work; *CSW*, Certified Social Worker; *DSW*, Doctor of Social Work; *LCSW*, Licensed Clinical Social Worker; *LICSW*, Licensed Independent Clinical Social Worker; *MSW*, Master of Social Work; and *PhD*, Doctor of Philosophy (in this case, in social work). *ACSW* refers to the Academy of Certified Social Workers.

Pastoral counselors are also trained in providing individuals with emotional support and guidance. Look for any of these credentials: *DDiv*, Doctor of Divinity; *DMin*, Doctor of Ministry; *MDiv*, Master of Divinity; and *PhD*, Doctor of Philosophy in his or her field of specialization.

A psychologist is specifically schooled in exploring the health of the mind. Applicable credentials include: *EdD*, Doctor of Education; *MA*, Master of Arts in Psychology; *PhD*, Doctor of Philosophy in his or her field of specialization; and *PsyD*, Doctor of Psychology.

It is important not to confuse the academic use of the term *doctor* with the medical use of the title. A *psychiatrist* is a medical doctor who specializes in psychological/mental health. If you are seeking a trained physician, you must select an *MD*, indicating medical doctor. He or she will have gone through the entire regimen and requirements of medical school, including board examinations, and will have accomplished full residency in psychiatry.

Additional helpful professionals include psychiatric nurses and mental health counselors. A practitioner who is a registered nurse is indicated by *RN*. You can request information concerning his or her experience in counseling. Also, some psychiatric nurses have studied through the graduate level in psychology. This will be indicated by an *MA*, signifying Master of Arts. Well-studied mental health counselors include those who have achieved an *MA* (Master of Arts) and/or an *MEd* (Master of Education) in their field.

WHAT PROFESSIONAL ORGANIZATIONS CAN I CONTACT FOR FURTHER INFORMATION?

American Academy of Pastoral Counselors
9504 A Lee Highway
Fairfax, VA 22031–2303
(703) 385–6967

American Psychiatric Association
1400 K Street, NW
Washington, DC 20005
(202) 682–6000

American Psychological Association
750 First Street, NE
Washington, DC 20002–4242
(800) 374–2721

National Association of Social Workers
750 First Street, NE, Suite 700
Washington, DC 20002–4241
(800) 638–8799

IS THERE AN AT-HOME TECHNIQUE I CAN USE?

Acknowledge and affirm that your pain can be related to your own negative thoughts and the anxious or angry reactions to events and stressors in your life. Make a promise to yourself that you will take control of this process by setting aside at least 15 minutes every day to be aware of what you are feeling and the consequent tension and/or pain in your body. Then, take a deep breath and release all the excess tension as you breathe out. Relax your muscles, returning your body to a less tense state. Your ability to process and release emotions, followed by a conscious effort to relax your muscles, will empower you to silence pain signals coming from your brain.

FELDENKRAIS METHOD

WHAT IS IT?

The Feldenkrais method teaches participants to become aware of movement patterns and to improve body motions, flexibility, posture, and breathing. This approach, which is particularly effective for chronic musculoskeletal problems, reprograms movement patterns to correct bad habits, alleviate pain, reduce stress, increase energy, and enhance self-image. The Feldenkrais method can be taught in either group or individual sessions.

The group sessions, called Awareness Through Movement, teach gentle and relaxing movements. The instructor leads the class through a series of simple exercises that are performed while sitting or lying down. These movements help to develop body awareness and increase mobility.

Individual sessions, called Functional Integration, offer one-on-one, intensive learning. The practitioner uses passive movement techniques and manually guides the student through body motions. The individual sessions are a process of learning conveyed by touch.

HOW DOES THE FELDENKRAIS METHOD VIEW THE PROBLEM OF SCIATICA?

The primary cause of most back problems is not using the supporting muscles of the body properly. Often times, in order to lessen pain or discomfort, people will alter the way they hold and move their bodies. These adjustments, which yield poor posture and improper movement, can become habitual and develop into symptoms of aches, pains, and muscle tightness. These symptoms can adversely affect the nervous system, including the sciatic nerve.

HOW DOES THE FELDENKRAIS METHOD TREAT SCIATICA?

The Feldenkrais method does not attempt to change the structure of the body through adjustments or manipulations. Rather, it instructs you to re-learn proper body movements by replacing old patterns of movement with new ones. By releasing unnecessary muscle tension brought on by poor habits, an easier, freer movement pattern is established in the body. This freer movement pattern can help to prevent injury and reduce stress-related illness, including sciatica.

The instructor may encourage you to imagine completing a movement before actually trying it. The idea behind this technique is that the body functions better with mindful preparation. If you select the group sessions, more complex movements will be introduced as classes progress, with the goal of helping you gain the confidence and ability to complete more challenging motions. You'll learn to move with greater ease, spontaneity, and freedom, resulting in benefits to the mind, the emotions, and the entire body. The mental and physical relaxation can ease the symptoms of sciatica.

Quick Tip

Driving can be uncomfortable for the individual with sciatica and/or other types of low back pain. It is best to position the seat so that it is as erect as possible and to move the seat closer to the steering wheel. You should reach the pedals without stretching. Press your low back firmly against the back of the seat and raise your knees slightly above hip-level. When driving for long distances, stop frequently and stretch; the vibrations from the road are tough on the spine.

IS THERE CURRENT RELEVANT RESEARCH?

To date, there are no studies published in the United States that directly study the Feldenkrais method's effect on sciatica symptoms. However, because the Feldenkrais method teaches awareness through movement, it is often helpful as part of the multi-disciplinary approach for individuals experiencing back pain, including sciatica.

WHAT IS THE ESTIMATED COST AND DURATION OF TREATMENT?

A personal Feldenkrais session generally costs $50 to $90 and lasts approximately 45 minutes. The long-term duration of this Functional Integration approach depends on you and the severity of your sciatica. Some individuals require weekly sessions over several months.

A group session—Awareness Through Movement—is less expensive, costing $8 to $15, yet also lasting for approximately 45 minutes. Some instructors offer drop-in classes. Others establish a set number of sessions, possibly requiring you to attend eight to twelve classes.

IS MY HEALTH INSURANCE LIKELY TO COVER THIS TREATMENT?

It is rare that the Feldenkrais method would be covered under your health insurance plan. However, if your health plan covers some form of complementary medicine, it would be best to contact the person in charge of the complementary medicine portion of the policy and speak to him or her directly regarding the specifics of coverage. Also, it is possible that your health plan covers complementary medicine and you are not aware of it. In either case, contacting your health-plan organization and speaking to a knowledgeable representative would yield the best results.

WHAT CREDENTIALS AND/OR EDUCATIONAL BACKGROUND SHOULD I LOOK FOR IN A PRACTITIONER?

In order for a practitioner to be certified in the Feldenkrais method, he or she must complete a four-year professional training program accredited by the Feldenkrais Guild. A practitioner who has been certified should have the following credential listed after his or her name: *GCFP*, indicating Guild Certified Feldenkrais Practitioner. These instructors are required to attend continuing education and to maintain active practices. This approach is a profession unto itself, but other healthcare professionals do incorporate it into their practices and can seek certification.

WHAT PROFESSIONAL ORGANIZATION CAN I CONTACT FOR FURTHER INFORMATION?

Feldenkrais Guild
524 Ellsworth Street, SW
Albany, OR 97321
(800) 775–2118

FOOT REFLEXOLOGY

WHAT IS IT?

The intricate structure of the foot and ankle consists of an extensive network of connective tissue, as well as numerous bones, muscles, joints, and nerves. With over 7,000 nerve endings in each foot, the feet provide an excellent source for neurological information. Foot reflexology is an approach that applies pressure to specific reflex areas on the feet in order to locate and correct problems in the body.

Practitioners of foot reflexology believe that specific reflex points on the feet correspond to particular areas and systems of the body. The goal of reflexology is to restore the natural flow of energy to these corresponding areas by stimulating certain areas on the feet. The practitioner applies stroking and sustained pressure (mostly with the thumb) to specific spots on the feet that reflect to the corresponding areas of the body where a problem originates. It is commonly believed that any patient experiencing nervousness or pain will respond well to the sensation of deep relaxation brought about by reflexology.

HOW DOES FOOT REFLEXOLOGY VIEW THE PROBLEM OF SCIATICA?

Practitioners of reflexology believe that energy flows through ten vertical lines that extend throughout the body from the toes to the head. Any energy blockage within these vertical lines can produce pain or disease in the areas corresponding to them. Sciatica is a result of such blockage. When a blockage occurs, waste-material granuals (uric acid and calcium crystals) accumulate around the corresponding reflex point of the foot, causing this point to feel tender to the touch.

HOW DOES FOOT REFLEXOLOGY TREAT SCIATICA?

The foot reflexologist will take note of any calluses, corns, swellings, deformities, tight areas, and the overall flexibility of the foot. He or she will stimulate specific points on the foot and assess the reaction

Quick Tips

Clothes may make the person, but they can also make back pain. Wearing tight, restrictive clothing that does not allow for flexibility can alter walking patterns, encourage poor posture, and impair proper body mechanics.

Footwear is not just a matter of fashion, either. Shoes with high heels create an exaggerated arch in the lumbar spine, forcing the weight of the body forward and leading to back strain. Quite differently, proper footwear not only provides protection and support for the feet, but also performs as a cushion and shock absorber for the spine.

to tenderness. Practitioners of this field are trained to assess health problems based on the tensions and sensitivities of the feet (extreme tenderness indicates a greater problem in that area). While holding the foot in a comfortable position, the reflexologist will apply pressure with the thumb and fingers to eliminate the tension and remove the waste products that have accumulated around the reflex point. Sciatic nerve impingement is generally indicated through tenderness in the middle of the heel or to the area just above and in back of the outside ankle bone. Most often, for the treatment of sciatica, these points are specifically worked upon.

The overall focus of reflexology for sciatica is to open up the blocked sciatic nerve pathway, relieve stress, and improve blood circulation, in order to remove waste products from the affected muscles. Throughout treatment, there should be clear communication regarding the comfort level of applied pressure. While techniques are gentle, there may be areas of the feet that are extremely sensitive or painful.

IS THERE CURRENT RELEVANT RESEARCH?

Results from a study originally published in the 1996 China Reflexology Symposium Report reported that of the 172 cases of sciatica studied, reflexology was significantly effective in 87 cases, and effective in 79. Only six people reported that they experienced no effect.

In total, this study reviewed the clinical application of 8,096 cases of various health conditions. In describing the results, "significantly effective" meant that all symptoms and signs disappeared upon completion of treatment, and that the disease did not recur in 3 to 6 months. "Effective" indicated the symptoms and signs disappeared, and after 3 to 6 months, symptoms did recur, but to a much lesser degree than prior to treatment. "No effect" meant there was no basic improvement of symptoms and signs, and that the disease recurred within 3 months after the treatment stopped.[1]

WHAT IS THE ESTIMATED COST AND DURATION OF TREATMENT?

Generally, a foot reflexology session costs $40 to $80 and lasts for 45 to 60 minutes. Results from this approach build over several treatments. Therefore, plan on attending a number of sessions.

IS MY HEALTH INSURANCE LIKELY TO COVER THIS TREATMENT?

It is rare that foot reflexology is covered by health-insurance plans. However, if your health plan covers some form of complementary medicine, it would be best to contact the person in charge of the complementary medicine portion of the policy and speak to him or her directly regarding the specifics of coverage. Also, it is possible that your health plan covers complementary medicine and you are not aware of it. In either case, contacting your health-plan organization and speaking to a knowledgeable representative would yield the best results.

WHAT CREDENTIALS AND/OR EDUCATIONAL BACKGROUND SHOULD I LOOK FOR IN A PRACTITIONER?

You should select a foot reflexologist that is designated as *Certified in the Original Ingham Method*. A certified practitioner is required to have completed a 200-hour program. This program includes 100 hours of documented clinical work. Also mandatory for certification is the successful completion of both a written and a practical exam. While foot reflexology is an independent field, various healthcare practitioners are certified in this approach and use it in their work.

WHAT PROFESSIONAL ORGANIZATION CAN I CONTACT FOR FURTHER INFORMATION?

International Institute of Reflexology
5650 First Avenue, North
St. Petersburg, FL 33710
(813) 343–4811

IS THERE AN AT-HOME TECHNIQUE THAT I CAN USE?

A convenient and effective way to massage the bottom of your feet—in particular, the heel portion—to help with sciatic pain is to place marbles in a shoe box and stand on them. Pressing and moving your foot over these marbles will stimulate the reflex points that are associated with the sciatic nerve.

HATHA YOGA

WHAT IS IT?

Hatha yoga is a gentle form of exercise training consisting of an array of body postures, slow movements, and proper breathing techniques. It is the most common form of yoga practiced in the Western Hemisphere today. The goal of Hatha yoga is to invigorate the body, clear the mind, and release the emotions. The yoga exercises provide gentle stretches that strengthen the back muscles and increase flexibility, as they build inner strength and a sense of body awareness. Because it is a gentle approach to healing the whole person, Hatha yoga is considered appropriate for everyone, including individuals with physical limitations.

HOW DOES HATHA YOGA VIEW THE PROBLEM OF SCIATICA?

Practitioners of yoga believe physical illness, such as sciatica, comes about when the body, mind, and spirit are not working together. They believe your mind has a profound influence on your physical body. A serene mind can help to produce a balanced, relaxed body, while a pattern of negative thoughts will ultimately create illness. Practitioners also believe that each person is born with a specific makeup or body type and this can have a significant influence on your state of health.

Often, people are faced with the challenge of working or living in an environment to which they do not adapt easily. For example, individuals who are most comfortable in quiet environments may find themselves working in high-stress, chaotic settings. When the body and mind are not in balance, a person may unconsciously manifest this imbalance through poor postural habits (such as slouching in a chair), unhealthy body mechanics, or a sedentary lifestyle and lack of exercise. As a result, many low back problems can develop, including sciatica.

HOW DOES HATHA YOGA TREAT SCIATICA?

Hatha yoga provides a balanced, disciplined workout that releases muscle tension, tones the internal organs, and energizes the mind, body, and spirit. Thus, natural healing can take place. A class, which may be large or small in number of participants, usually begins with breathing exercises and then turns to stretching and toning techniques.

Proper breathing techniques train the body and mind to relax, to be more aware of and better able to release any build-up of tension in the muscles. Breathing and posture exercises promote physical and emotional health by restructuring and toning the supporting muscles of the back and abdomen, as they address the psychological aspect of low back pain, as well. Then, as you perform various postures that incorporate bending your body forward and bringing your head toward your knees, you will stretch your back muscles and lengthen your spine. This helps to create stability, to realign the spine, and therefore improve overall posture. Improved posture means a healthier environment for the spinal nerves, including the sciatic nerve.

The exercises of Hatha yoga consist of slow twisting movements that improve mobility, tone the spinal column muscles, and ease lower back pain. They support the muscles of the back evenly, not only to improve posture and body mechanics, but also to increase flexibility and joint range of motion. There are various levels of Hatha yoga. You should start with a beginner's class and move up in diffi-

> ## Quick Tip
>
> When stretching, you should feel the stretch in the muscle, not in the joint. Joints cannot be stretched, so if you feel the stretch in the joint area, you are probably stretching ligaments that connect muscles to joints. Ligaments are more likely to tear than to stretch.
>
> Remember to always stretch slowly; never *bounce* into a stretch. Bouncing stimulates the myotatic stretch reflex—a muscle-protective mechanism—making it more likely that you tear the muscle, rather than stretch it.

culty until you find the appropriate level. Expect a little soreness at first, as your body gets used to the stretching and toning. But the increased muscle strength, spinal realignment, and relaxation that are the end product of a commitment to Hatha yoga can diminish sciatica discomfort.

IS THERE CURRENT RELEVANT RESEARCH?

Researcher LaForge conducted a study on Hatha yoga in 1997. The conclusion was that Hatha yoga programs can reduce anxiety, improve self-confidence, and improve muscular strength.[1] These benefits are important factors in the relief of sciatica.

WHAT IS THE ESTIMATED COST AND DURATION OF TREATMENT?

Generally, a Hatha yoga class costs $10 to $20 and lasts for 60 to 90 minutes. The program will extend over a number of weeks, possibly involving eight to ten classes. Results from Hatha yoga are gradual; this approach has a cumulative effect. To get the most out of Hatha yoga, it is important to practice the techniques regularly.

IS MY HEALTH INSURANCE LIKELY TO COVER THIS TREATMENT?

Some health plans cover for Hatha yoga, but the parameters of coverage vary. If you know that your health plan covers some form of complementary medicine, it would be best to contact the person in charge of the complementary medicine portion of the policy and speak to him or her directly regarding the specifics of coverage. Also, it is possible that your health plan covers complementary medicine and you are not aware of it. In either case, contacting your health-plan organization and speaking to a knowledgeable representative would yield the best result.

WHAT CREDENTIALS AND/OR EDUCATIONAL BACKGROUND SHOULD I LOOK FOR IN A PRACTITIONER?

Yoga instructors are trained by yoga masters over a number of years. There is no official certification program. You will have to rely on rec-ommendations and on your own evaluation of the instructor. We sug-gest that you try one introductory class for evaluation purposes, to find out if you are comfortable with the instructor and the level of the program. During this session, you can inquire about the instructor's experience and talk to other participants who are familiar with the instructor's techniques. The most important factor in choosing a Hatha yoga teacher, however, is how much of a positive connection you, personally, feel under his or her guidance.

Hatha yoga is a discipline unto itself. However, certified aerobics instructors often incorporate the stretches and other aspects of Hatha yoga into their aerobics classes. In addition, Hatha yoga programs are available on videotape for at-home instruction. These options offer two other ways in which to benefit from Hatha yoga techniques.

WHAT PROFESSIONAL ORGANIZATION CAN I CONTACT FOR FURTHER INFORMATION?

International Association of Yoga Therapists
20 Sunnyside Avenue, Suite A243
Mill Valley, CA 94941
(415) 332–2478

IS THERE AN AT-HOME TECHNIQUE THAT I CAN USE?

The *cat stretch* helps bring necessary nutrients to the spine, while increasing flexibility. Get down on your hands and knees. Gently allow your back to sink, bringing your abdomen towards the ground.

Now round your back towards the ceiling. Hold the position for 5 seconds. Repeat the cat stretch ten times.

MASSAGE

WHAT IS IT?

Massage is the practice of kneading or otherwise manipulating a person's muscles and other soft tissue with the intent of improving that individual's well-being. It is a natural way to relax and relieve tired, sore muscles. The human skin is the body's largest sensory organ. The second layer of skin (dermis) contains sensitive receptors that pick up and send messages to the brain when stimulated by touch.

The main goal of massage is to accelerate the healing of soft tissue injury, improve circulation, and decrease tension and pain. This is accomplished by increasing joint range of motion and flexibility, stretching connective tissue, decreasing inflammation, and releasing endorphins.

HOW DOES MASSAGE VIEW THE PROBLEM OF SCIATICA?

It is commonly believed that a pinched nerve can be caused not only by a herniated disc, but also by trauma to soft tissue (skin, connective tissue, muscles, ligaments, joints). Muscle strain is an example of such trauma. When unnecessary tension is placed upon the supporting muscles of the lower back, muscle strain can occur. A sedentary lifestyle, obesity, poor posture, and lack of exercise are all contributing factors to poor muscle function. A strain usually occurs after improperly lifting, twisting without stretching, or trauma to the lower back. When tight muscles press against and irritate the sciatic nerve, a burning, stabbing pain with numbness and weakness may occur. The pain radiates across the lower back and occasionally into the buttock region.

Heavy exercise technically causes soft-tissue trauma, albeit the long-term effects are worth it. During heavy exercise, stressed muscles develop tiny ruptures called micro-traumas. To protect these torn areas, the muscle cells and, therefore, the injured area swell with fluid. The inflamed cells not only push painfully against nerves, such as the sciatic nerve, but they also reduce circulation and slow the healing process.

Sciatica can also be caused by weak abdominal and/or lower back muscles. When these muscles are weak, they cannot adequately hold the spine erect, making the pinching of a nerve more likely. The sciatic nerve is particularly susceptible to such pressure.

HOW DOES MASSAGE TREAT SCIATICA?

The focus of massage therapy is to reduce pressure on the nerves by lengthening the connective tissue, improving the muscle tone, reducing stress, and interrupting the pain-spasm-pain cycle. There are various forms of massage. Below, we briefly describe two forms that can aid in the relief of sciatica.

Sports massage is a form of soft-tissue mobilization that is geared toward athletes and participants of leisure sports who suffer from injuries such as major pulls, tears, strains, stiffness, pain, and/or sore spots. This type of massage is also effective for those who want to prevent the loss of mobility, enhance athletic performance, increase endurance, and maintain good health and physical conditioning. Sports massage is usually confined to a specific area and is seldom given to the full body. It is typically used to break down scar tissue and/or to spread muscle fibers, allowing for increased blood flow. The improved circulation that results brings more oxygen and nutrients to the tissue, allowing for a healing response to take place.

Quick Tip

The backpack is no longer simply a piece of camping equipment; countless people use backpacks as school bags, shopping bags, and general carry-alls. To avoid back problems, the weight of the backpack should be evenly distributed between the two shoulders. If you carry your backpack on one shoulder, remember to periodically switch it from shoulder to shoulder, to prevent additional stress on the muscles of the shoulders, neck, and back.

Inflammation ultimately decreases and fluid is carried away via the bloodstream. Lymph circulation is improved, as well. This permits loosened wastes and toxins to washed away.

Swedish massage combines modern principles of anatomy and physiology with traditional Oriental practices of massage. It aims to manipulate soft tissue in muscle by using the fingers and/or palms. Swedish massage is generally applied to the full body. Practitioners of Swedish massage perform numerous techniques that improve blood flow to the muscle and skin, stretch connective tissue, tone muscles, reduce anxiety, and release endorphins. Because it is used widely, variations in practitioner techniques are common. Some techniques involve light massage strokes, to increase circulation to the skin, while others use deeper strokes that increase bloodflow in the arteries and stimulate movement of lymphatic fluid throughout the body. An example of a technique is the practitioner's application of finger pressure to the lumbar area of your spine, increasing blood flow to the muscles in this area and removing tension. This allows a healthier environment for the sciatic nerve. As occurs during sports massage, the increase in circulation that results from a Swedish massage allows for a greater amount of oxygen to nourish the cells and aids in washing away toxins.

Additional techniques of Swedish massage may employ any of the following: kneading; rolling; gentle compression; quick and steady shaking; and light tapping. Massage used to relieve sciatica with muscular components to the pain would concentrate on breaking up muscle spasms and increasing the flow of oxygen to the muscles. Lengthening and relaxing muscle groups would also be part of the treatment. Specifically, trigger point pressure may be applied to the center of the buttock region for a maximum of 20 seconds, monitoring the change in pain on the trigger point on a scale from one to ten. Other trigger points in the buttock area may also be located and treated in the same way.

Cross fiber friction massage could be used on the sacroiliac joints—the two areas on the low back (sacrum) where the low back connects to the hip bones. This technique involves thumb pressure, which the practitioner uses across the muscle fibers at a 90° angle; the goal is to separate the muscle fibers and break down the adhesions that stick the fibers together. Also, proprioceptive neuromuscular facilitation (PNF)—a process of progressively stretching and relaxing muscles of the body—around the area of the sciatic nerve may be used. If helpful, massage would be performed down the legs to increase the circulation of blood. Swedish massage is very beneficial to the health of the skeletal, muscular, circulatory, nervous, respiratory, digestive, and urinary systems.

IS THERE CURRENT RELEVANT RESEARCH?

The Touch Research Institute (TRI), formally established in 1992, is devoted solely to the scientific study of touch and its applications in the fields of science and medicine. Under the direction of Tiffany Field, PhD, TRI's distinguished team of researchers explores the connection between touch therapy and the effective treatment of disease. The Institute has ongoing studies on back pain. Although not specific to the pain of sciatica, results are relevant because they have shown that massage therapy reduces anxiety, back pain, and sleep disturbances, and also improves mood.[1] These benefits are essential when seeking relief from sciatica.

WHAT IS THE ESTIMATED COST AND DURATION OF TREATMENT?

Generally, a massage session costs $45 to $80 and lasts from 30 to 60 minutes. The frequency of massage sessions, the duration of treatment, and even the duration of individual sessions depends on your preferences and your needs. One session can be effective in terms of relaxation and acute pain. However, sciatica is generally a chronic condition, so relief most often requires a regular massage schedule.

IS MY HEALTH INSURANCE LIKELY TO COVER THIS TREATMENT?

Some health plans cover for massage therapy, but the parameters of coverage vary. If your health plan covers some form of complementary medicine, it would be best to contact the person in charge of the complementary medicine portion of the policy and speak to him or her directly, regarding the specifics of coverage. Also, it is possible that your health plan covers complementary medicine and you are not aware of it. In either case, contacting your health-plan organization and directly speaking to a knowledgeable representative would yield the best results.

WHAT CREDENTIALS AND/OR EDUCATIONAL BACKGROUND SHOULD I LOOK FOR IN A PRACTITIONER?

Credentials for massage therapists depend on the type of massage and the state in which the therapist desires to practice. To obtain certification, a massage therapist must complete a training program in general massage from a school accredited by the American Massage Therapy Association/Commission on Massage Training Accreditation (AMTA/COMTA) and/or the State Board of Education. In order to practice sports massage, once the above-described requirement has been fulfilled, the practitioner is eligible to complete additional training from the AMTA National Sports Massage Certification Program. If this process is completed, the instructor will designate his or her training with the initials *CSMT*, indicating Certified Sports Massage Therapist.

The most common credential for massage therapy is *CMT*, indicating Certified Massage Therapist, and *LMT*, signifying Licensed Massage Therapist (in states that have licensing available). We recommend that you seek a massage therapist who, in addition to either of the above accomplishments, carries the *NCTMB* credential, referring to National Certification in Therapeutic Massage and Bodywork. You may also see the following: *CMP*, Certified Massage Practitioner; *LMP*, Licensed Massage Practitioner; and *MT* or *MsT*, Massage Therapist. There is no difference between a practitioner and a therapist. Generally, a massage professional is referred to as a massage therapist, and complementary care professionals are referred to as practitioners.

WHAT PROFESSIONAL ORGANIZATION CAN I CONTACT FOR FURTHER INFORMATION?

American Massage Therapy Association
820 Davis Street, Suite 100
Evanston, IL 60201
(847) 864–0123

National Certification Board for Therapeutic Massage and Bodywork
8201 Greensboro Drive, Suite 300
McLean, VA 22102
(703) 610–9015

Aromatherapy

The power of aroma is evident through its capacity to affect the emotions and the body. Aromatherapy uses the aromatic, essential oils from herbs and flowers, assigning them as therapeutic treatments. Your sense of smell is connected to the part of your brain that controls the autonomic (involuntary) nervous system. As a result, you respond immediately and involuntarily to scent. The powerful perfume of the essential oils stimulates the release of neurotransmitters in your brain. These brain chemicals can have effects that are calming, sedating, pain reducing, stimulating, or euphoriant.

There are several methods of inhalation that can be used to disperse the aroma. Most simply, drops of oil can be placed on a handkerchief or in steaming hot water. The scent will travel through the environment. Also, the diffuser method is very effective; a diffuser is a device that, when heated, spreads the vapors throughout a room. In addition, spritzing from a spray bottle into the air will disperse the aroma. Finally, soaking in a therapeutic bath allows both inhalation and absorption.

When essential oils are applied to the skin in specially prepared lotions, they can serve as antibacterial, anti-inflammatory, and astringency agents. Some massage practitioners apply prepared lotions that contain diluted oils directly to the skin during treatments. This method allows you to benefit not only from the aroma, but also from the absorption of the oils into the skin. Practitioners believe these oils are carried throughout the body via the bloodstream, and can strengthen and heal muscle tissue, joints, and organs.

The following essential oils are beneficial for the relief of sciatica: clary sage; German chamomile; lavender; and sweet marjoram. They contain properties that are both anti-spasmodic and sedative. Therefore, they assist in relieving nervous tension (which often causes muscular aches and pains), as well as in reducing muscle spasms and inflammation.

MEDITATION

See *Relaxation/Meditation*, pages 93 to 101.

MYOTHERAPY

WHAT IS IT?

Myotherapy is a manual form of deep pressure massage that focuses on trigger points—tender, congested spots on muscle tissue that radiate pain to other areas of the body. In fact, this approach is sometimes referred to as trigger point therapy. Practitioners of myotherapy apply pressure to these locations in order to relieve tension, relax muscle spasms, improve circulation, and decrease pain. The goal of this pressure is to interrupt the interior signal that is causing the trigger point and the resulting pain. Then the therapist essentially reprograms the signal through relaxing stretching exercises.

Myotherapy is beneficial for a number of muscle-related conditions, particularly low back pain. It is not a cure for diseases, but rather a means to relieve pain and accelerate the healing process.

HOW DOES MYOTHERAPY VIEW
THE PROBLEM OF SCIATICA?

A trigger point marks an area of injury or insult to a muscle. It can develop as a result of a fall, poor posture, or over-exertion. Once a trigger point is established in the body, it can be activated at anytime by physical or emotional stress. When a trigger point sends a muscle into spasm, the body responds by putting more muscles into spasm, creating a pain-spasm-pain cycle. Sciatica is understood as the result of a pain-spasm-pain cycle that was caused by the stimulation of a trigger point along the pathway of the sciatic nerve. The signals need to be interrupted in order for the body to discontinue the progression of deep, sharp, and disabling pain.

HOW DOES MYOTHERAPY TREAT SCIATICA?

A practitioner of myotherapy will press along the length of a muscle to locate a trigger point. This process can be painful, but with good dialogue between you and your practitioner, it can be brief. For sciatica sufferers, the buttocks area is the place where trigger points are most often found. Once a trigger point is located, the therapist will apply pressure directly to it for several seconds using knuckles, fingers, or elbows, and then slowly release. You can expect to feel immediate relief after the applied pressure. The pressure breaks the pain-signal pattern that is being communicated between the brain and the muscle.

After the successful interruption of the pain signal, the muscle relaxes. The myotherapist then passively stretches the muscle. The neuromuscular system (which includes nerves that control muscle function) uses this new information to reorganize, thus relieving tension, back pain, and restrictions. Myotherapy can decrease the swelling and stiffness associated with back pain, as well as increase range of motion, flexibility, and coordination.

In addition, the myotherapist will teach you a series of exercises that will help keep the muscles in your low back pain-free. Common symptoms of people suffering with sciatica are tight hamstrings and weak abdominal muscles. Exercises that gently stretch and strengthen muscles are generally recommended to relax and fortify these areas. Sciatica patients are also taught to avoid pain-producing posture, so that they can avoid the recurrence of trigger points.

Quick Tip

If moving a heavy object such as a piece of furniture, *push, don't pull.* When you push an object, you can use your legs and body weight, which helps to take pressure off the low back.

IS THERE CURRENT RELEVANT RESEACH?

The Touch Research Institute at the University of Miami Medical Center, under the direction of Tiffany Fields, PhD, is conducting ongoing studies on the effects of trigger point therapy (or myotherapy) for pain relief. No definitive results are currently available, but the Touch Research Institute provides a newsletter of their work and a website for updated information.[1] See the References section of the book, under "Myotherapy."

WHAT IS THE ESTIMATED COST AND DURATION OF TREATMENT?

Generally, a myotherapy session costs $45 to $80 and lasts for 30 to 60 minutes. While acute attacks may be relieved in one session, sciatica is often a chronic condition and, therefore, is likely to require repeated treatments. This is true even taking into consideration the practice of at-home techniques.

IS MY HEALTH INSURANCE LIKELY TO COVER THIS TREATMENT?

Some health plans cover for myotherapy, but the parameters of coverage vary. If your health plan covers some form of complementary medicine, it would be best to contact the person in charge of the complementary medicine portion of the policy and speak to him or her directly regarding the specifics of coverage. Also, it is possible that your health plan covers complementary medicine and you are not aware of it. In either case, contacting your health-plan organization and speaking to a knowledgeable representative would yield the best results.

WHAT CREDENTIALS AND/OR EDUCATIONAL BACKGROUND SHOULD I LOOK FOR IN A PRACTITIONER?

Practitioners of myotherapy should be certified. Certification involves a 9-month, 1,400-hour training program, a board examination, and 45 hours of continuing education credits every other year. A myotherapist designates certification with the *CBPM* credential, indicating Certified Bonnie Prudden Myotherapist.

You may select a practitioner whose practice is exclusive to myotherapy, as myotherapy is an independent approach. However, various healthcare practitioners in other fields may also incorporate the techniques of myotherapy into their work. So you may be able to gain the benefits of myotherapy from these professionals as well.

WHAT PROFESSIONAL ORGANIZATION CAN I CONTACT FOR FURTHER INFORMATION?

Bonnie Prudden Pain Erasure
7800 E. Speedway
Tucson, AZ 85710
(800) 221–4634

International Myotherapy Association
2200 Hamilton Street
Allentown, PA 18104
(610) 437–6187

IS THERE AN AT-HOME TECHNIQUE THAT I CAN USE?

Four different stretching exercises for the low back are described below. They provide relief from the pain associated with low back conditions, including sciatica.

Exercise 1

- Lie on your back, with your arms at your side and your legs bent at the knees.

- Grab hold of your left knee with your two hands and pull your leg towards your chin. Your head should be bent forward to increase the stretch. The right leg remains bent. Hold this position for 8 seconds.

- Rest your head on the floor. The right leg remains bent. Release the left knee and straighten the leg out. Hold the outstretched leg about twelve inches above the floor for 8 seconds.

- Return to position 1 and begin again, alternating legs. Repeat the exercise three or four times on each side.

Exercise 2

- Lie on your right side, knees slightly bent.

- Pull your left knee towards your chest and hold for 8 seconds.
- Bring the left leg back to starting position, but hold about 10 inches above the right leg for 8 seconds.
- Lower the leg and repeat the exercise three or four times.
- Repeat the entire sequence with the opposite leg.

Exercise 3

- Lie on your stomach, with your head resting on your arms.
- Tighten your stomach and butt muscles. Hold for 8 seconds.
- Repeat this exercise three or four times.

Exercise 4

- Lie on your back, with your knees bent and your feet shoulder width apart.
- Push your stomach up, slightly arching your back. Your shoulders and butt should remain touching the floor.
- Now bring your stomach down, tightening your stomach muscles as you press the low back firmly into the floor. Hold for 8 seconds.
- Repeat this exercise three or four times.

NUTRITIONAL COUNSELING

WHAT IS IT?

It is commonly believed that good health is directly related to eating a balanced diet. What we *should* eat and what we *do* eat are rarely the same. Many factors, from lifestyle and time constraints to culturally learned eating habits, determine our diets. Furthermore, societal pressure to look a certain way can make eating a psychological nightmare rather than an enjoyable approach to good health. Nutrition, though, is fundamental to well-being and generally is a common denominator in every condition treated.

Nutritional counseling covers a wide range of assessments and dietary philosophies. Nutritionists offer education on numerous subjects, including facts about food items, eating patterns, vitamin/mineral intake, food allergies, and weight loss. They work with clients to design individual diets that provide both variety and proper nutrition. The promotion of wellness thorough dietary and lifestyle recommendations can be a primary or adjunct therapy.

HOW DOES NUTRITIONAL COUNSELING VIEW
THE PROBLEM OF SCIATICA?

In today's fast-paced and stressful world, it is easier to eat for convenience rather than to eat for health. But the body requires the proper nutrients in the proper amounts in order to promote tissue maintenance and strong supporting muscles. Without good nutrition, the back and its associated nerves are as likely as any other part of the body to become susceptible and weak. Poor postural habits, unhealthy body mechanics, athletic injury, and tight muscles from emotional trauma can all put additional stress on the support muscles of the back.

Muscle strain is a major contributing factor in low back pain and the development of sciatica. When muscles are regularly worked, they produce byproducts such as lactic acid. A buildup of lactic acid accumulating in the muscle can cause irritation, leading to pain. This buildup of lactic acid can become worse by dehydration and the regular consumption of highly processed junk food containing insufficient nutrients. Other factors such as deficient mineral and vitamin intakes can lead to weak bones, low energy, poor muscle development, and unhealthy nerves.

Quick Tip

When lifting objects such as laundry baskets or grocery bags, always bend your knees and keep your back straight. Hold the objects close to the body and lift by primarily using the arm, leg, and abdominal muscles. The farther away you hold an object, the more pressure you put on your vertebrae. Holding the object close to you distributes the weight over the length of the spine, pelvis, and legs.

HOW DOES NUTRITIONAL COUNSELING TREAT SCIATICA?

Nutritional counseling designs a good nutritional regimen, beginning with a planned diet that will provide the body with an adequate supply of the nutrients necessary to function properly and maintain health, including spinal health. In order to draw up an individualized plan, the practitioner will first determine any nutritional deficiencies and food allergies that you might have. He or she does so through a medical history evaluation, which includes medication, current diet, present back symptoms, emotional state, energy level, and exercise habits. Nutritional deficiencies and allergic reactions to certain foods may also be determined through a skin test or through hair or urine samples.

After the nutritionist has assessed your dietary needs, he or she provides you with a nutritional program. A diet that regulates caloric intake and helps maintain a healthy weight is quite beneficial for a painful low back. So if you are carrying extra weight, the nutritionist may put you on a low-calorie regimen. Mineral and vitamin nutritional supplements may be recommended for deficiencies, in order to increase energy and maintain good health. Strengthening the body with proper nutrition is a natural way to take control of your life, to increase the quality of life, and to maintain optimal body functioning. Sciatica symptoms can be reduced as a result of these improvements.

IS THERE CURRENT RELEVANT RESEARCH?

A study presented by Robert A. Lillo, MD, at the annual meeting of the American Medical Society for Sports Medicine, described a case study of a middle-aged woman who suffered with symptoms of sciatica for over 14 months. She spent thousands of dollars on numerous diagnostic tests, to no avail. The woman was eventually diagnosed as vitamin-B_{12} deficient. She received vitamin-B_{12} injection therapy and her condition rapidly improved. Ultimately, the woman made a steady recovery. It was emphasized that a vitamin-B_{12} deficiency can have a devastating effect on the spinal cord.[1]

WHAT IS THE ESTIMATED COST AND DURATION OF TREATMENT?

Generally, a session with a nutritional counselor costs $50 to $80 and lasts for 30 to 60 minutes. Professionals within the field of nutrition most often require their clients to attend three or more office visits. Then additional sessions may be scheduled for further instruction on integrating a particular nutrition regimen into daily life.

If the nutrition counselor recommends supplements, there will be additional expenses. Luckily, vitamins, minerals, and food supplements are available in health food stores, drugstores, apothecaries, supermarkets, and mail-order catalogs. Ask your nutritional counselor to recommend quality brands that are reasonably priced.

IS MY HEALTH INSURANCE LIKELY TO COVER THIS TREATMENT?

Many insurance companies provide insurance coverage for nutritional counseling when prescribed by a physician and performed by a registered dietician or certified nutritional consultant. Call your health-plan representative to find out parameters for your specific policy.

WHAT CREDENTIALS AND/OR EDUCATIONAL BACKGROUND SHOULD I LOOK FOR IN A PRACTITIONER?

There is a variety of programs and schools that train nutritional counselors. A nutritional counselor should have one of the following titles: *CNC*, Certified Nutritional Consultant (accredited by the American Association of Nutritional Consultants); *LD*, Licensed Dietitian (state license); *ND*, Doctor of Naturopathic Medicine; *RD*, Registered Dietitian (accredited by the American Dietetic Association).

Practitioners of Ayurvedic medicine and practitioners of Traditional Chinese Medicine can also offer legitimate nutritional counseling. Ayurveda is an ancient system of medicine that was developed in India over 5,000 years ago. It promotes the maintenance or attainment of optimal health through the use of a combination of approaches, such as exercise, herbal remedies, massage, meditation, and nutritional counseling. The United States has established no licensing procedures or accrediting boards for Ayurvedic practitioners. Those who study Ayurveda can consult with clients, but cannot practice as medical doctors. If you seek a practitioner of Ayurvedic medicine, select one who has completed his or her full medical degree in India and holds a *BAMS,* indicating a Bachelor of Ayurveda Medical Studies. Also, some healthcare practitioners complete a 1-year certification program and are very capable of counseling on Ayurvedic nutritional techniques.

Those who are trained in Traditional Chinese Medicine should list one of the following after their names: *DOM/OMD,* Doctor of Oriental Medicine; *MOM,* Master of Oriental Medicine. Like Ayurvedic medicine, this is also a multi-disciplined system of medicine, involving many approaches.

WHAT PROFESSIONAL ORGANIZATION CAN I CONTACT FOR FURTHER INFORMATION?

American Dietetic Association
216 West Jackson Boulevard, Suite 800
Chicago, IL 60606–6995
(800) 366–1655

American Association of Nutritional Consultants
810 South Buffalo Street
Warsaw, IN 46580
(888) 828–2262

American College for Advancement in Medicine
P.O. Box 3427
Laguna Hills, CA 92654
(800) 532–3688

IS THERE AN AT-HOME TECHNIQUE THAT I CAN USE?

The following are recommendations from James F. Balch, MD, and Phyllis A. Balch, CNC, who are experts in the field of nutrition and the authors of *Prescription for Nutritional Healing* (Avery Publishing Group, 1997):

• While you are experiencing sciatica and/or other back problems, avoid meat and all products that contain animal protein. The uric acid in animal products puts strain on the kidneys, and this strain can add to back pain, including sciatica.

- Completely avoid gravies, oils, fats, sugar, or rich or highly processed foods.

- Drink two 8-ounce glasses of water (of good quality) *as soon as you feel the pain begin.* Relief is felt within minutes of this natural remedy. Why? Because dehydration is frequently a culprit behind muscle aches and back pain. In order to prevent acidic wastes from accumulating in the tissues of the body, you need to drink a minimum of eight 8-ounce glasses of water every day.[2]

OSTEOPATHY

WHAT IS IT?

Osteopathy is a type of medicine that is based on the following beliefs: the entire body needs to be considered when treating a condition, and the musculoskeletal system plays a key role in any dysfunction. This approach addresses physical, psychological, and lifestyle factors when determining the underlying cause of a condition. A doctor of osteopathy (DO) primarily uses manipulation of the musculoskeletal system to restore healthy body structure, relieve pain, promote optimal mobility and flexibility, as well as improve overall health. These practitioners frequently endorse other forms of complementary care and adhere to the notion that the body, if cared for properly, is capable of healing itself.

HOW DOES OSTEOPATHY VIEW THE PROBLEM OF SCIATICA?

Sciatica is looked upon as a disturbance in the musculoskeletal system. This system, which includes bones, joints, muscles, ligaments, and connective tissue, plays a significant role in the well-being of the other systems of the body. Poor postural habits (sitting in a slouched position) and unhealthy body mechanics (lifting heavy objects incorrectly), physical trauma (sports injuries), and emotional trauma (life stressors) can all effect the musculoskeletal system. An insult to this system can result in injury or the buildup of lactic acid, leading to pain.

A pain signal is sent from the area of trauma to a section of the spinal column that supplies the nerves to that area. The nerves from the spinal column send back a protective impulse to the muscles to tighten up, creating a further decrease in flexibility and circulation, as well as an increase in pain. Sciatica can result when the back muscles are traumatized and contracted and/or the spinal structures are mis-aligned.

HOW DOES OSTEOPATHY TREAT SCIATICA?

The goal of osteopathic treatment for sciatica is to increase mobility, improve circulation, decrease muscle and ligament tension, and decrease pain in the low back region and along the sciatic pathway. This is brought about through the manipulation of the joints and soft tissue, and through exercise to improve poor posture and body mechanics.

The practitioner of osteopathy assesses your posture and identifies areas of stiffness on the spine. An examination and evaluation of various joints will be performed to assess immobility and the origin of the pain. Vertebrae mobilization, which involves gently massaging the area around the vertebrae, is performed to relax tight muscles near the area of pain and those affected by the sciatic nerve. But a gentle form of general massage is used prior to mobilization of the vertebrae, to prepare the injured area. Often, relaxation exercises are taught for home use, in order to prevent the recurrence of back pain.

Quick Tip

Whether shoveling snow or digging dirt, pick up small amounts and keep the loaded shovel close to your body. Remember to bend at the knees, not at the back.

IS THERE CURRENT RELEVANT RESEARCH?

A survey of fifty clinical experts on low back pain was taken to assess the perceived clinical effectiveness of complementary/alternative therapies for four defined categories of low back pain. It was published in the *Journal of Manipulative Physiological Therapy* in February,

1999. For acute, uncomplicated low back pain, osteopathy (and chiropractic) were rated as effective by most experts.[1]

WHAT IS THE ESTIMATED COST AND DURATION OF TREATMENT?

If paying out-of-pocket, an osteopathic treatment may cost $80 to $95. However, osteopathy is covered under most health plans. Parameters vary considerably. The number of necessary visits and the duration of treatment will also vary greatly, depending on the cause and severity of your sciatica.

IS MY HEALTH INSURANCE LIKELY TO COVER THIS TREATMENT?

Osteopathic treatment is covered under most health plans, but the parameters, such as the number of visits allowed and the amount of co-payments, if any, will vary. Coverage for osteopathic treatment is handled much like that for outpatient visits to a primary care physician.

WHAT CREDENTIALS AND/OR EDUCATIONAL BACKGROUND SHOULD I LOOK FOR IN A PRACTITIONER?

A Doctor of Osteopathy, indicated by *DO*, undergoes the same duration and intensity of training as a medical doctor. Practitioners attend 4 years of training at an osteopathic college, after receiving their Bachelor's Degree, and then go on to complete internships and residencies.

WHAT PROFESSIONAL ORGANIZATION CAN I CONTACT FOR FURTHER INFORMATION?

American Osteopathic Association
142 East Ontario Street
Chicago, IL 60611
(800) 621–1773
(An operator will refer you to your state osteopathic association, which in turn will provide a list of osteopathic physicians in your area.)

Craniosacral Therapy

The origins of craniosacral therapy can be found in the work of Sutherland, who was a student of osteopathy. The craniosacral system includes: the bones of the cranium (skull, face, and mouth); the spine and sacrum (the lower end of the spine); the membranes that connect the cranium to the sacrum, and the cerebrospinal fluid—the clear fluid that circulates through and around the brain and spinal cord. Craniosacral therapy uses gentle, hands-on techniques to treat stress and obstructions in this area that can lead to low back pain. Osteopaths may use craniosacral therapy as one of their techniques.

Each person has a palpable craniosacral rhythm. A trained practitioner can feel this subtle movement when his or her hands are placed on the cranium. The rhythm results from the expansion and contraction caused by the increase and decrease of cerebrospinal fluid, which is produced and re-absorbed at a regular rate. This rhythm is similar to those produced by the heart and by the rate of respiration.

It is commonly believed that during infancy, particularly during the birth process, when the bones of the skull are alterable, compression on the skull can lead to future injuries. Practitioners of craniosacral therapy maintain that the suture lines connecting the bones of the skull never close completely, and they respond in a small degree to changes in pressure of the cerebrospinal fluid. These changes can lead to emotional and physical problems. The approach aims to release tension not only at the various points where the craniosacral bones meet, but also on the meninges, which are the membranes of the cerebrospinal area.

The practitioner usually helps to reestablish balanced rhythm and normal function by applying gentle pressure to the cranium with his or her hands. This pressure creates subtle manipulations that allow a release of tension along the cranial sutures, the meninges, and in response, the entire craniosacral region. Relaxing musculature and restoring fluid movement can bring greater health to the spinal column, ultimately providing a healthier environment for the sciatic nerve.

American College for Advancement in Medicine
P.O. Box 3427
Laguna Hills, CA 92654
(800) 532–3688

PERSONAL TRAINING

WHAT IS IT?

Personal training is a combination of fitness assessment, fitness instruction, and motivational techniques that help the client achieve physical conditioning goals. A personal trainer will design a unique program specifically for the individual. Motivation is often the primary factor when starting a new exercise program or when continuing an exercise program on a regular basis. Thus, motivation and positive reinforcement are emphasized, in addition to proper body mechanics and the correct forms of breathing when exercising.

Exercise sessions stress endurance, strength, and flexibility, while focusing attention on personal goals and interests. It is important that the client enjoys the exercise program, believes in its benefits, and follows guided instruction, so that he or she will be willing to continue with the regimen. Of primary importance for those suffering with low back pain are exercises that lengthen the spine and stretch tight muscles. Often, physical activity programs will be tailored to particular back problems.

HOW DOES PERSONAL TRAINING VIEW THE PROBLEM OF SCIATICA?

Low back problems, particularly sciatica, are frequently associated with lack of flexibility, poor posture, and excess body weight (gained in the abdominal area) often brought about through sedentary lifestyle and lack of exercise. It is widely believed that when back and abdominal muscles are not regularly stretched, they tend to shorten and become inflexible. This lack of flexibility can leave these muscle groups weak and without the ability to hold the spine erect, particularly when these muscles are needed for rotation of the spine during normal activities.

Quick Tip

A pull-up bar can provide an excellent source for pain relief when your back suddenly becomes tight and is on the verge of going into spasm. The pull-up bar, conveniently placed in a doorway, must be well secured. When your back is about to go into spasm, firmly grasp the bar and lower yourself by slowly bending your knees. Your feet should not be completely off the ground. Hold this position for 20 seconds and slowly return to standing position. Now repeat. This will provide a degree of weightlessness and a relieving stetch for your back.

Lack of flexibility in the lumbar spine makes the low back vulnerable to injury leading to irritation of the sciatic nerve. It can also encourage poor posture and subsequently result in abnormal muscular tension, joint and ligament strain, as well as irritation to vertebral discs. And in response to excess weight in the abdominal area, the body pulls forward, forcing the supporting muscles of the back to increase their workload to maintain stability, balance, and proper posture. Stress on the supporting muscles of the back puts additional pressure on the lumbar discs.

HOW DOES PERSONAL TRAINING TREAT SCIATICA?

When developing an exercise program to eliminate the symptoms of sciatica, a routine that increases the flexibility of spine's joints, as well as increasing the length and strength of the abdominal and back muscles, is recommended. Activities that help reduce muscle tension and pain, such as flexion exercises (knees to chest) and exercises that round and arch the low back, are frequently used.

When the large muscle groups of the body are exercised, the brain produces chemicals (endorphins) that serve as the body's natural pain killers. Endorphins not only decrease pain, but also help reduce tension and increase the sense of well-being. Exercises can involve stretching, cardiovascular and endurance training, and weight training, using proper body mechanics under close supervision. Stretching exercises are an excellent warm up to cardiovascular activities, as they increase flexibility and range of motion for all of the joints. Cardiovascular workouts and endurance training help reduce body fat, decrease stress and tension, and enhance the circulatory system's ability to supply oxygen to the tissues. Walking is a great cardiovascular activity that activates all of the large muscle groups. Prior to walking, be sure to perform hamstring and low back stretches, and avoid hill workouts once your walk has begun. Walking up a hill can tighten hamstring muscles, which may impinge on the sciatic nerve. Finally, weight training builds muscular strength to help the body withstand the activities of daily living and to prevent injuries. It also develops muscle tone, endurance, and replaces fat with muscle.

During personal training, any physical activities that reinforce poor postural habits are not performed. Sports such as running, jogging, golf, bowling, tennis, and certain swimming strokes should be avoided unless you reeducate yourself to avoid improper posture and movement that may have led to the original back injury. Also, while exercise can be very beneficial for problems in the low back area, the benefits can be lost within a few weeks if exercise stops. It is frequently recommended to continue a minimal exercise program rather than to stop exercising once the problem has subsided.

IS THERE CURRENT RELEVANT RESEARCH?

Back in the 1960s, Swedish physician Alf Nachemson developed an instrument that measures the load on a person's lower spine while standing. He discovered that this load amounts to more than half of a person's body weight. Keeping this statistic in mind, it is clear that maintaining a healthy body weight and physical condition can greatly reduce the amount of pressure on the lower spine.

A study was published in *Orthopedics* in 1995 demonstrating the effect of exercise on individuals with chronic low back pain. The average length of symptoms prior to the study was 26 months. Of the 627 patients completing the exercise program under study, 76 percent of them reported excellent or good results. In a follow-up one year later, 94 percent of those with excellent or good results maintained their improvements.[1]

Studies recently published at Tufts University have shown that weakness and frailty problems can start as early as age forty, but they are not inevitable or irreversible. Establishing a regular fitness program allows for prevention of these problems in young people, and improved strength and activity levels in older adults.[2] Increasing your overall fitness will, in turn, promote a healthy spinal environment, including a proper pathway for the sciatic nerve.

The National Institutes of Health's Office of Medical Applications of Research and the National Heart, Lung and Blood Institute convened a Consensus Development Conference on Physical Activity and Cardiovascular Health. While this panel focused on the relationship between physical activity and cardiovascular health, the panel's studies also relate to physical activity and low back pain, which would include sciatica. The panel found that physical inactivity is widespread among Americans of all ages. This inactivity results in weight gain, inflexibility, a decrease in necessary nutrients to the spine, and increased pressure on the lumbar spine due to long periods of sitting. It was concluded that children and adults should engage in 30 minutes of moderate-intensity physical activity on most, and preferably all, days of the week.[3]

WHAT IS THE ESTIMATED COST AND DURATION OF TREATMENT?

Generally, a personal training session costs $40 to $60. The duration of individual sessions, the frequency of sessions, and the duration of the entire treatment approach vary greatly, depending on specific goals and fitness levels, as well as the severity of the sciatica.

IS MY HEALTH INSURANCE LIKELY TO COVER THIS TREATMENT?

Some health plans offer discounted membership rates at affiliated health clubs, YMCA's, and hospital wellness centers. It is best to contact your policy representative to find out with what clubs, if any, your specific plan is associated.

WHAT CREDENTIALS AND/OR EDUCATIONAL BACKGROUND SHOULD I LOOK FOR IN A PRACTITIONER?

Personal trainers should successfully complete a 20- to 24-hour course on personal fitness training/education, counseling, and exercise physiology. The course can be taken either over a number of weeks or at an intensive weekend seminar. Documentation on having passed a written and practical examination at the end of the course is necessary. In addition, after completing the certification training, personal trainers have the option of taking a national certification examination through the Aerobic and Fitness Association of America (AFAA). Re-certification through the completion of continuing education units is required every two years, in order to maintain a current certification status.

WHAT PROFESSIONAL ORGANIZATION CAN I CONTACT FOR FURTHER INFORMATION?

American Council on Exercise
5820 Oberlin Drive, Suite 102
San Diego, CA 92121
(800) 234–9229

IS THERE AN AT-HOME TECHNIQUE THAT I CAN USE?

Staying in shape and maintaining a healthy body weight by participating in regular exercises and/or activities are extremely beneficial to the health of your back, as well as your emotional health. But if you suffer from sciatica, try to avoid activities that place excessive force and twisting on your spine. Such movements are common during golfing, tennis, skiing, and weight lifting. Actually, even with activities that are considered therapeutic for the low back, such as swimming, running, and bicycling, precautions should be taken. Below are some tips on performing these activities in a healthier manner.

Golf—Generally, the body rotates and bends while extending to swing. To avoid injury, warm up slowly on the practice range. In particular, stretch the lower back. Be careful to use proper form, correct body mechanics, and appropriate playing clubs for your body type.

Tennis—During the quick stop-and-go actions of a tennis game, the body is likely to twist. To avoid problems, stretch before starting your

---

Quick Tip

If you must stand for long periods of time, prop one foot on any object. This will take pressure off your low back. Change your position often. Stretch, bend, or lean against a wall, if possible.

---

game, warm up slowly, and rally before play. Be aware of and maintain good playing form.

Skiing—During skiing, the body experiences quick twisting of the spine. To avoid injury, strengthen your legs, increase the flexibility of your body, and always use correct form.

Weight Lifting—The back is forced into unhealthy arches if you use weights that are too heavy. And while lifting any heavy weight, your body experiences excessive bending and twisting. For a healthier routine, warm up before lifting and slowly build up to heavier weights. Be sure to use proper body mechanics, and make it an exercise goal to increase your flexibility, as this will help your body respond better to lifting weights.

Swimming—Avoid the breast stroke and crawl stroke because they force the lumbar spine to arch. Swim slowly and increase duration gradually.

Running—Avoid running on hard surfaces, as well as running up hills. The pounding of the hard surface can stress joints and the hills can tighten hamstrings, putting additional tension on already-tight back muscles. To avoid stress on lower back muscles, run frequently but go shorter distances.

Bicycling—When cycling, bike adjustments are needed to prevent low back strain. First, there should be two inches of space between the top bar and your crotch when you are standing with feet on ground. Next, the seat should be adjusted so that your leg is nearly fully extended when the bottom pedal is closest to the ground. The front of the seat should be slightly tipped upward. Also, straight handlebars are best for upright sitting. They should be positioned just below the top of the bike seat. And finally, wider tires help lessen road vibration to the spine.

In summary, if you are a committed participant in any of these sports and want to continue, remember to always complete warm-up exercises before beginning play. Warming up will increase blood circulation to your ligaments and muscles. Stretching your lower back before and after playing can loosen tight muscles and prevent further injury. Always maintain good posture, proper playing form, and the appropriate body mechanics.

PSYCHOTHERAPY

See *Emotional Pain Relief Therapy,* pages 46 to 54.

QIGONG

WHAT IS IT?

The ancient Chinese believed that universal life energy—*chi*—is present in every living creature. This energy is said to circulate throughout the body along specific pathways called *meridians.* Qigong, an ancient Chinese method of healing, is movement therapy geared toward developing and improving the circulation of internal and external chi. It consists of breathing exercises, meditation, and stretching techniques. Many forms of the martial arts have developed from qigong. However, the focus of qigong is steeped more in healing than in self-defense.

Derived from Buddhist, Taoist, and Confucian philosophies and based on the instinctive movements of animals, qigong promotes strength, balance, and overall well-being. The exercises involve: gentle, rhythmic, swinging postures; stretching movements; meditation; and deep relaxation breathing. The slow movements will foster a meditative state of quietness and help to calm the emotions and the mind. The exercises are easy to learn and are suitable for all ages. They will become more effective and more natural with practice.

HOW DOES QIGONG VIEW THE PROBLEM OF SCIATICA?

As long as chi flows freely, health is maintained. If, however, the energy current becomes blocked, the system is disrupted and pain and illness occur. When the flow of chi is interrupted or blocked particularly in the kidney, bladder, or gallbladder meridians, which are associated with the low back, sciatica can result.

HOW DOES QIGONG TREAT SCIATICA?

Qigong is generally taught in a class environment where individuals gain the skills and abilities to practice on their own. Movements are designed to avoid the tightening of muscles and the stressing of joints, and to encourage concentration on the energy flow within the body. The goal of qigong is to develop an awareness of chi's presence and movement through techniques that bring the body into a relaxed, flexible state. Concentration on and sensitivity to the flow of the body's energy is taught through a technique that involves remaining motionless for an extended period of time (anywhere from a few minutes to an hour). Then the slow-paced exercises stretch every ligament and tendon, move every joint, and flex every muscle.

The regular practice of qigong exercises leads to an improvement in circulation, balance, and flexibility, as well as an increase in range of motion. Furthermore, these exercises improve overall relaxation and awareness, and generally promote good health by encouraging a slower pace, a gentler appreciation of the body, and a clearer awareness of the self. By strengthening and moving the essential energy of the body and enabling it to flow without obstruction, sciatica can be treated and health can be maintained.

Quick Tip

When retrieving a small object from the floor, reduce your risk of further back pain by resisting the urge to bend solely at the waist. Whether bending your knees to a full squat or half-way, it is important to keep your feet shoulder-width apart and your knees in line with the tops of your feet.

IS THERE CURRENT RELEVANT RESEARCH?

Numerous research studies have been conducted, primarily in China, on the medical applications of qigong. A 1996 article by Sandler that reviewed selected studies on the medical applications of qigong indicated that chronic conditions such as hypertension, aging, and neuromuscular problems are showing promise in benefiting from the practice of qigong.[1] These chronic conditions can have direct effects on the onset and/or severity of sciatica.

WHAT IS THE ESTIMATED COST AND DURATION OF TREATMENT?

Generally, a personal qigong session costs approximately $60, while a group session costs $10 to $20. The class lasts for 45 to 60 minutes. You are likely to achieve feelings of relaxation and well-being during the very first class. However, we recommend that you make a commitment to a series of qigong sessions, in order to truly learn proper movements and to gain the maximum benefit from this approach.

IS MY HEALTH INSURANCE LIKELY TO COVER THIS TREATMENT?

It is rare that qigong is covered under health insurance plans. However, if your health plan covers some form of complementary medicine, it would be best to contact the person in charge of the complementary medicine portion of the policy and speak to him or her directly, regarding the specifics of coverage. Also, it is possible that your health plan covers complementary medicine and you are not aware of it. In either case, contacting your health-plan organization and speaking to a knowledgeable representative would yield the best results.

WHAT CREDENTIALS AND/OR EDUCATIONAL BACKGROUND SHOULD I LOOK FOR IN A PRACTITIONER?

At the present time, there is no official certification for practitioners of qigong. Those who serve as qigong instructors have studied under qigong masters. Your best evaluation tool is to attend an introductory class. During this session, you can assess whether or not you are comfortable with the instructor and the level of the course. The most important factor is to find an instructor with whom you are able to make a positive connection.

WHAT PROFESSIONAL ORGANIZATION CAN I CONTACT FOR FURTHER INFORMATION?

American Oriental Bodywork Therapy Association
Laurel Oak Corporate Center, Suite 408
1010 Haddenfield-Berlin Road
Voorhees, NJ 08043
(609) 782–1616

RELAXATION/MEDITATION

WHAT IS IT?

Relaxation and meditation techniques involve deep breathing exercises, muscle relaxation, and focused attention, all of which work toward shutting down the anxiety-producing fight-or-flight response of the body. The fight-or-flight response is the body's reaction to a perceived threat, resulting in a buildup of stress hormones. Relaxation and meditation can reduce heart rate, blood pressure, breathing rate, and brain wave-patterns. The resulting state is helpful for physical and emotional healing.

Many people integrate spirituality or particular religious practices into their relaxation or meditation programs. Some of the reported experiences include: peacefulness; serenity; calmness; a sense of well-being; selflessness; a connection to a higher being; and an altered state of consciousness. The regular practice of relaxation/meditation can decrease anxiety, alleviate symptoms of stress and disease, prevent future disorders, and provide a strong sense of purpose and a renewed level of energy.

HOW DOES RELAXATION/MEDITATION VIEW
THE PROBLEM OF SCIATICA?

Stress often occurs when the continuous demands of life overwhelm our abilities to cope with them. The body's response to a stressful situation is to release chemicals into the bloodstream, such as epinephrine and cortisol. Epinephrine has the physical effect of increasing blood pressure and heart rate, while cortisol inhibits the immune system. A stressful situation will also increase the production of lactic acid, resulting in muscle tension. Emotional symptoms, such as tension, anger, anxiety, and the inability to concentrate are further complications brought about by the excess of stress.

It is generally believed that stress can play a major role in the progression of an illness. Stress can be either a direct cause or a contributing factor to low back problems, including sciatica. As muscles experience chronic tension and posture and body mechanics suffer, the alignment of the spine is likely to be compromised. The pathway of the sciatic nerve may thus be obstructed or distorted, and the nerve itself may become compressed and irritated.

HOW DOES RELAXATION/MEDITATION TREAT SCIATICA?

Your reaction to tension is a learned response, and you always have the option to learn a new behavior. Fortunately, through relaxation, the body is able to reverse many of the long-term effects brought on by undue stress. By relaxing the body and the mind, muscle tension and spinal pressure are reduced, spinal alignment is improved, and the symptoms of low back pain, including sciatica, can be alleviated.

Although each person's experience with relaxation or meditation will be unique, the basic goal is to find a system that helps to clear the mind of interfering thoughts and, thereby, to relax the body. Find a technique and a body position that allows you to remain comfortable throughout the process. Sitting is often suggested, but other possible positions are kneeling, squatting, sitting in the lotus position (cross-legged on the floor), or lying down. Finally, close your eyes. With these basic principles in place, breathing techniques and muscle relaxation begin.

Slow, deep breaths are encouraged as you are instructed to clear your mind and/or progressively relax different parts of your body. If you practice on your own, you can train yourself by repeating certain breathing patterns and by disciplining yourself to return to a state of clear-minded focus. Many people choose to be guided at first, so that they can become proficient at the patterns that will relax the body. A multitude of techniques are used, some of which are discussed below.

Biofeedback is performed by a practitioner and uses a simple electronic monitoring device. You are connected to the device by electrodes adhesively attached to the skin surface. These electrodes collect information on vital body functions such as heart rate, blood pressure, muscle tension, brainwave activity, and skin temperature. The process is painless. Data registers within the biofeedback machine and is changed into signals. These signals can be heard as sounds (beeps), seen as video images (flashes), or monitored by dial readings. They act as feedback, helping you to become more aware of changes in your body.

The biofeedback practitioner instructs you to alter or slow down the signals through the use of relaxation, meditation, and/or visualization. Deep breathing exercises and focusing on positive images may be used. Ultimately, biofeedback enables a person to gain psychological control over physiological processes. The goal is to maintain the acquired skills of relaxation even when the biofeedback device is no longer used.

Christian meditation, often called contemplation, is a process of quieting the mind with the intention of becoming more fully aware of God, the teachings of Christianity, and the self. Prayer is used to further the meditative state. In fact, within a number of religious traditions, prayer is a form of meditation in itself, since the process of prayer generally involves taking time from normal routine to calm the mind and to focus on faith in a higher power.

Through *guided imagery/visualization,* you and your therapist work to find mental pictures that will stimulate natural healing responses. You may use your own imagery or work with visualizations suggested by the therapist. The images/visualizations help to alleviate anxiety and to bring about changes in attitude and behavior. They encourage you to work through emotions connected with trauma, illness, or other life circumstances. Therapists will often teach visualization exercises as self-help tools that you can use outside of therapy.

Hypnotherapy is an approach during which the therapist guides the client into a trance-like state called *hypnosis*. It is a state between sleep and waking, referred to as the alpha level, in which you are relaxed and capable of intense concentration. This state can be induced through several simple techniques, among which are verbal suggestions and having you observe a continuously moving object.

In the hypnotic state, you become relaxed and open to suggestions for change. Hypnotherapy is a powerful therapeutic tool that can remove resistance to an open and honest exploration of the consciousness. The left hemisphere of the brain governs the conscious mind, particularly language and logic. The right hemisphere, encompassing the unconscious mind, is associated with emotions and synthesis—the ability to pull it all together. Hypnotherapy allows communication between both sides.

Progressive muscle relaxation fosters awareness of muscular tension in every part of the body, and teaches methods to release that tension. It generally begins with calming breathing exercises and mental focus activities that promote serenity. Next, each individual part of the body, from the toes to the scalp, is flexed (tensed) and then released with notions of weightless and floating. The result is a wave of relaxation that eventually covers the entire body.

Siddha meditation involves repeatedly reciting short words or phrases—a *mantra*. This promotes focus and relaxation. The sound helps to free the mind from distracting thoughts and provides a vibrating frequency that brings on the state of meditation. Breath control and breath awareness are also part of this technique.

Stress management techniques can help you to cope more effectively with stress, so that the negative effects on the body, mind, and emotions can be reduced. Stress results from the normal, everyday pressures of living. Financial concerns, work obligations, and raising children are common stressors. Life stage transitions, such as marriage, divorce, births, deaths, illness, moving, starting a new job, and unemployment, also create much anxiety and tension. Stress management training combines education on the sources and effects of stress, discussions of your particular stress reactions, and instructions in helpful coping skills.

Transcendental meditation, like Siddha meditation, involves the use of the mantra—short words or phrases that are repeated for relaxation/meditation purposes. However, unlike Siddha meditation, the mantra is repeated in the mind, not recited aloud. This is done while sitting in a comfortable position and with your eyes closed. The goal is to achieve a deep, inner level of consciousness and relaxation.

It is evident that there are a number of valuable relaxation and meditation techniques that will encourage greater health in your body and your mind. Try different techniques until you find one that really works for you. The process will become more effective with practice. Therefore, it is best to make a commitment to regular relaxation/meditation sessions.

Quick Tips

If falling asleep is difficult, try some of these pampering strategies. Take a warm bath right before climbing into bed. Fill your room with the aroma of lavender; essential oils can be used in the form of room spritzers or heated on a light bulb using a lamp ring. Listen to quiet music and release the tension of the day with deep abdominal breaths, in and out.

Find a comfortable position in which to sleep. Avoid sleeping on your abdomen and sleeping on your back with legs fully extended. If you want to sleep on your back, place pillows under your knees. The best position is side-lying (fetal position) with a pillow under your neck and head, and a pillow between your knees.

IS THERE CURRENT RELEVANT RESEARCH?

The National Institutes of Health formed an assessment panel on the integration of behavioral and relaxation approaches for the treatment of chronic pain and insomnia. The panel used a four-point scale that ranked the evidence as strong, moderate, fair, or weak. The panel concluded that the evidence was strong for the effectiveness of relaxation techniques in reducing chronic pain in a variety of conditions. Sciatica would fall under the category of chronic pain. Hypnosis and biofeedback were also determined effective in the treatment of chronic pain. It was not concluded, however, that any one technique is consistently more effective than another. This distinction can only be made on an individual level, according to a person's own preferences.[1]

WHAT IS THE ESTIMATED COST AND DURATION OF TREATMENT?

Obviously, there are many methods of relaxation and meditation, some of which can be done on your own. However, it is beneficial to have some formal, guided instruction if you desire to make a serious commitment to a specific technique (with the exception, of course, of personal prayer). Some techniques actually require certified or licensed practitioners.

A biofeedback session generally costs $50 to $150 and lasts for approximately 50 minutes. The large range of cost is due to variations in the education and credentials of the practitioners. The number of necessary treatments that you will need depends on the severity of your sciatica and your individual response.

A session of hypnotherapy will generally cost $40 to $150 and lasts for 30 to 50 minutes. The long-term duration and the frequency of your treatment is very individualized, depending on your particular condition and goals. A wide variety of professionals use hypnotherapy, and therefore, the fee range is large.

Meditation instructors are generally trained under masters of these techniques. Individual sessions cost anywhere from $40 to $150 and last for 30 to 90 minutes, depending on the specific discipline and the instructor. A group session is less expensive, generally costing $15 to $35 and lasting for 60 minutes. One session may prove effective as an introduction, and then can be followed up with at-home audiotapes. Even though techniques can be self-taught, for maximum benefit, you should enroll in at least one to three group or individual sessions, in order to become better skilled at the techniques. Private instruction is often a part of psychotherapy, but can be arranged as needed with a practitioner.

IS MY HEALTH INSURANCE LIKELY TO COVER THIS TREATMENT?

Relaxation/meditation training completed under the guidance of a licensed psychotherapist, social worker, psychologist, or psychiatrist is covered under most health plans, but the parameters vary. Contact your health plan organization for the specifics of coverage.

WHAT CREDENTIALS AND/OR EDUCATIONAL BACKGROUND SHOULD I LOOK FOR IN A PRACTITIONER?

For biofeedback, seek a practitioner who has been certified through the Biofeedback Certification Institute of America; look for *BCIAC* after his or her name, indicating Biofeedback Certification Institute of America Certified. There is no state licensing. Various healthcare practitioners use biofeedback and other relaxation techniques in their practices, including some psychiatrists, psychologists, social workers, nurses, physical therapists, occupational therapists, speech therapists, exercise physiologists, chiropractors, dentists, and physician's assistants. Look for the appropriate credentials of these practitioners according to the requirements of their specific professions.

If selecting a meditation instructor, your best tool of evaluation is to attend a session and assess how comfortable you are with the instructor. There are no set credentials for these healing techniques, as instructors learn from masters. The main criteria is that you feel safe with your instructor and that you are able to attain a positive connection with each other. You should find his or her guidance effective in helping you to attain a release of stress and tension.

For hypnotherapy, we recommend that you choose a practitioner who has a professional license in one or more of the healing arts, such as a psychiatrist, psychologist, social worker, nurse, pastoral counselor, physician, or dentist, and who holds additional approval as a certified hypnotherapist, indicated by the initials *CH*. This credential means that the practitioner has completed a hypnotherapy training program approved by the American Board of Hypnotherapy, or has passed an examination approved by this board, or has maintained a private or group practice in hypnotherapy for 3 years.

WHAT PROFESSIONAL ORGANIZATIONS CAN I CONTACT FOR FURTHER INFORMATION?

General Information

American Association of Pastoral Counselors
9504 A Lee Highway
Fairfax, VA 22031–2303
(703) 385–6967

American Psychiatric Association
1400 K Street, NW
Washington, DC 20005
(202) 682–6000

American Psychological Association
750 First Street, NE
Washington, DC 20002–4242
(800) 374–2721

National Association of Social Workers
750 First Street, NE, Suite 700
Washington, DC 20002–4241
(800) 638–8799

Specific Techniques

Association for Applied Psychophysiology and Biofeedback
10200 W. 44th Avenue, Suite 304
Wheat Ridge, CO 80033
(303) 422–8436

Biofeedback Certification Institute of America
10200 W. 44th Avenue, Suite 304
Wheat Ridge, CO 80033
(303) 420–2902
E-mail: bcia@resourcenter.com; include your local zip code, and the institute will send you a list of certified practitioners in your area.

American Board of Hypnotherapy
16842 Von Karman Avenue, Suite 475
Irvine, CA 92606
(800) 872–9996

American Society of Clinical Hypnosis
2200 East Devon Avenue, Suite 291
Des Plaines, IL 60018
Send a 33¢-stamped, business-size, self-addressed envelope for a state listing.

National Guild of Hypnotists
P.O. Box 308
Merrimack, NH 03054
(603) 429–9438

Transcendental Meditation
(888) 532–7686
This number will ring in the state from which you are calling. The operator will provide you with information on transcendental meditation instructors near you.

IS THERE AN AT-HOME TECHNIQUE THAT I CAN USE?

The next time you get upset, stop for a moment and feel the emotions in your body. Pay attention to the extra tension in your muscles, become aware of your body posture, then take a deep breath and release all the excess tension as you breathe out. Relax your muscles, returning your body posture to a less tense state.

ROLFING

WHAT IS IT?

Rolfing is a form of structural integration that involves deep manipulation of the connective tissue in order to restore the body's natural alignment. The practitioner performs manipulations with the fingers, thumbs, forearms, and elbows. Practitioners of Rolfing believe that the structure of the body affects both physical and mental health. They further believe that gravity plays a key role in healthy body structure and if the body is properly aligned, it can work harmoniously with gravity and maintain a natural state of health and flexibility.

The agenda of the practitioner is to systematically treat the entire body in a series of ten sessions. During the treatments, clients are taught to synchronize their breathing along with the manipulations. This should contribute to the process of restoring proper posture and realigning the body.

HOW DOES ROLFING VIEW THE PROBLEM OF SCIATICA?

The alignment of our bodies often can be distorted by the way we sit, stand, walk, or sleep. And as we adapt to unhealthy positions, poor posture becomes habitual. We find diminished motivation to change the patterns that eventually lead to movement restrictions and chronic pain.

When the body is put under this continuous stress, the connective tissue (which covers all muscles) hardens, bunches, and loses its flexibility. The easy, free movements of the body gradually become restricted. Over time, this added workload can effect the body's natural vertical alignment and breathing patterns, creating a loss of vitality, as well as a decrease in flexibility. Low back pain, including that of sciatica, can thus develop as a result of injury, from weak muscles and lack of flexibility; poor posture, from a continuous battle with gravity; or emotional distress.

HOW DOES ROLFING TREAT SCIATICA?

Rolfing practitioners apply deep, slow pressure to soften and lengthen connective tissue, layer by layer. By stretching and lengthening the connective tissue, the surrounding tissue can be restored to its proper function and the body is put into proper alignment with gravity. Each Rolfing session focuses on the manipulation of the connective tissue in one area of the body. During this process, the waste and toxins that have become embedded in the surrounding soft tissue are loosened and carried away. The result is increased movement ability, proper postural alignment, and a reduction in low back pain.

IS THERE CURRENT RELEVANT RESEARCH?

No studies have assessed Rolfing methods specifically for the treatment of sciatica, but present research considerations indicate the Rolfing is a viable approach for further study in the relief of back pain. For example, a study on Rolfing was conducted at the UCLA Department of Kinesiology in 1977. It found that individuals who experienced Rolfing showed improvements in posture and displayed more energetic body movements with increased flexibility.[1]

A study published by Cottingham in 1988 examined the effects of

Quick Tips

Household activities, if not performed carefully, can put tremendous stress on your back and cause significant pain. Follow these tips for safer movement:

When ironing, stand tall and do not lean over the ironing board. If possible, rest one foot on a stool or a box and alternate legs often. Do not lean your body into the leg that is holding you up.

When sweeping, again, stand tall. Hold the broom close to your body. Take advantage of the length of the broom so that you are not bending over it. Alternate the hand that is on top and also the side of the body along which you are holding the broom.

When vacuuming, let the vacuum do the work; avoid using unnecessary pressure. Maintain a straight body and don't lean over the vacuum. With an upright vacuum, it is best to hold the handle close to your hips and, if possible, to alternate the side on which you hold the vacuum. If your vacuum has a separate motor, squat and reposition the machine, instead of pulling on the hose.

soft tissue manipulation (Rolfing method) on thirty-two young, healthy men who had anteriorly tilted pelvises—that is, their pelvises tilted toward the front of the body. Such a tilt can cause spinal stress and dysfunction. The subjects were randomly assigned to an experimental and a control group. After a 45-minute session, one of the observations noted was that the experimental group (who had the soft tissue manipulation) showed a significant decrease in the pelvic-tilt angle, when compared with the control group. This study provided theoretical support for the Rolfing method of soft-tissue pelvic manipulation when it comes to certain types of low back dysfunction and musculoskeletal disorders associated with anxiety-induced muscle problems.[2]

In a case study outlined in the *Journal of Orthopaedic and Sports Physical Therapy* and reviewed in *Massage Magazine*, a nineteen-year-old woman with low back pain for two years was given an integrative treatment approach of Rolfing and the Alexander Technique. The study was conducted over a six-session period. The first three sessions were devoted to Rolfing and the last three were used for the Alexander Technique. Results showed a significant decrease in the woman's low back pain compared to the temporary relief received from previous regimens of rest, massage, and chiropractic. The article noted that the outcome of the study cannot be used as evidence for the validity of the approaches, but that the results could stimulate research for these approaches when dealing with chronic back pain.[3]

WHAT IS THE ESTIMATED COST AND DURATION OF TREATMENT?

Generally, a Rolfing session costs $75 to $125 and lasts for 60 to 90 minutes. The same fee is set for each session, and you may be charged a single fee for the ten-session program. The cost of this treatment is dependent on the individual practitioner and varies widely.

IS MY HEALTH INSURANCE LIKELY TO COVER THIS TREATMENT?

Some health plans provide coverage for Rolfing, but the parameters of coverage vary. If your health plan covers some form of complementary medicine, it would be best to contact the person in charge of the complementary medicine portion of the policy and speak to him or her directly regarding the specifics of coverage. Also, it is possible that your health plan covers complementary medicine and you are not aware of it. In either case, contacting your health-plan organization and speaking to a knowledgeable representative would yield the best results.

WHAT CREDENTIALS AND/OR EDUCATIONAL BACKGROUND SHOULD I LOOK FOR IN A PRACTITIONER?

There is an established certification program for the practice of Rolfing; the practitioner must complete an 18-week training program at the Rolf Institute. Plus, a 7-week introductory course in anatomy, physiology, and kinesiology is given as a mandatory prerequisite to this program. You can identify whether a practitioner has had this training by looking for the initials *CR,* indicating Certified Rolfer, after his or her name.

There is also an advanced certification program. For this extra credential, a Rolfer is required to have a minimum of 3 years experience in active practice, must take 18 continuing education units through the Rolf Institute, and pass a 6-week course at the same school. The following credentials signify this advanced training: *ACR,* Advanced Certified Rolfer; or *CAR,* Certified Advanced Rolfer.

WHAT PROFESSIONAL ORGANIZATION CAN I CONTACT FOR FURTHER INFORMATION?

Rolf Institute
205 Canyon Boulevard
Boulder, CO 80306
(800) 530–8875

TAI CHI

WHAT IS IT?

Tai chi is an ancient Chinese movement therapy. It consists of a traditional series of slow, graceful movements that are intended to unite the mind and body, to build inner strength, and to create and develop a healthy flow of energy—*(chi)*—within the body. Breathing techniques are combined with meditation and a routine of slow, calculated movements. By moving at a decelerated pace, your body's habitual responses are challenged. You are forced to re-evaluate every movement. This makes you more aware of the body's energy, and more in control of your own well-being.

HOW DOES TAI CHI VIEW THE PROBLEM OF SCIATICA?

Like other approaches that stem from Traditional Chinese Medicine (TCM), the philosophy behind tai chi is that sciatica occurs when there is an obstruction in the free flow of chi. Wind, cold, or damp can invade the body and cause blockages along the *meridians*—the pathways along which chi flows. This can create pain and illness anywhere in the body. Sciatica is attributed to obstruction in either bladder, gallbladder, or kidney meridians, which are associated with the lower back. If cold is the cause, the sciatic pain will be more intense.

In addition, obstruction of chi can be due to improper positioning and movement, and even to lack of proper mindfulness in dealing with everyday stresses. Tension, whether mental or physical, can trigger reactions in the muscles that create back pain and related problems, including sciatica. Therefore, learning to relax and restore proper movement to the body is important.

HOW DOES TAI CHI TREAT SCIATICA?

The smooth exercises of tai chi cause joints to open, chronic energy blocks to dissolve, and chi to circulate throughout the body. Relaxed posture and circular movements encourage limberness, thus helping to release tension. The combination of turning, stretching, and twisting allow every part of the body to be exercised without strain. The slow movements foster a meditative state of quietness and help to clear the mind of distracting thoughts.

When flow of chi is restored, the healing process begins. Furthermore, circulation is improved to areas of the body that were suffering from strain and pressure, nourishing the areas with more oxygen. Toxins are carried away and greater well-being is experienced.

Tai chi's ability to rejuvenate, rather than exhaust, makes it a valuable exercise program for the relief and prevention of back pain. This exercise system requires little muscular strength, but entails much concentration and discipline. Though the slow movements of tai chi seem simple, it takes time to learn the proper motions and coordination. Breathing must be synchronized with the precision of the movements. The soft flowing movements become more effective and natural with practice.

IS THERE CURRENT RELEVANT RESEARCH?

A randomly assigned, controlled study was conducted to assess the effectiveness of tai chi on "pain, mood and disability in patients with chronic low back pain" over a 6-week period. The study involved eleven of the twenty standard tai chi moves. Ninety-minute sessions were held only once a week. Also, participants were instructed to practice tai chi for at least 15 minutes daily. Pain was measured at the starting point, at three weeks, and then at six weeks. Researchers found that compared with the control group (who did not perform tai chi), participants who practiced tai chi had significant reductions in pain. The concluding data supported the "primary hypothesis that 6 weeks of tai chi reduces pain intensity in individuals with chronic low back pain compared with routine care."[1] Sciatica can be included among the sources of chronic low back pain.

WHAT IS THE ESTIMATED COST AND DURATION OF TREATMENT?

Generally, a tai chi class costs $10 to $15 and lasts for 60 minutes. An alternative option is to purchase an instructional videotape, which is an economical way to learn tai chi. To get the most out of the practice of tai chi, it is important to study this healing system over a considerable period of time.

IS MY HEALTH INSURANCE LIKELY TO COVER THIS TREATMENT?

While tai chi can certainly contribute to physical and psychological well-being, it is not formally recognized as a medical treatment by health insurance companies. Therefore, you are not likely to receive any coverage for tai chi classes.

WHAT CREDENTIALS AND/OR BACKGROUND SHOULD I LOOK FOR IN A PRACTITIONER?

There are no certification or licensing procedures for tai chi instructors at the present time. Those who seek to teach tai chi study under tai chi masters over long periods of time. Your best tool of evaluation is to attend an introductory class. During this session, assess how comfortable you are with the instructor and the level of the class. Also, talk to other students who have experienced the teacher's techniques. The most important thing to look for is a very positive connection between you and the instructor.

WHAT PROFESSIONAL ORGANIZATION CAN I CONTACT FOR FURTHER INFORMATION?

American Oriental Bodywork Therapy Association
Laurel Oak Corporate Center, Suite 408
1010 Haddenfield-Berlin Road
Voorhees, NJ 08043
(609) 782–1616

TRAGER APPROACH

WHAT IS IT?

The Trager approach is a form of movement re-education. The practitioner uses a series of gentle, rhythmic, rocking and shaking movements, along with rotation and traction of the limbs, to loosen the joints, increase mobility, and release chronic patterns of tension. The practitioner supports and moves the limbs in a manner that promotes flexibility and provides pain relief. These gentle movements put the client into a deep state of relaxation. No oil or lotions are required, nor is pressure or deep tissue manipulation needed to create structural change.

This is a learning technique aimed at correcting movement dysfunction. Practitioners provide appropriate physical and verbal cues during sessions, helping the client to re-learn healthier movement patterns. The practitioner creates within the individual a sense of how it feels to be able to move freely and without pain. The client's role is to remain passive and relaxed.

The Trager approach has no rigid procedures; movements are adjusted to the individual so that when muscle tightness is located, the practitioner can ease the tension and re-establish a sense of easy, free movement. Because of the dramatic increase in mobility that results from this treatment, even after one session, people with low back pain or severe movement restrictions generally experience great improvement.

HOW DOES THE TRAGER APPROACH VIEW THE PROBLEM OF SCIATICA?

Practitioners of the Trager approach believe that the mind and body are not separate from each other. They believe that low back pain, in all probability, has a physical origin and needs to be treated with physical intervention, but also that psychological problems affect low back pain and need to be addressed. Adverse circumstances such as poor posture, stress, emotional traumas, illness, and unhealthy body mechanics cause deep-rooted psychological and physiological patterns. Such patterns can cause low back pain, including the pain associated with sciatica, resulting in the inability to move the spine and pelvis in a free and easy fashion.

Quick Tip

If you have a low back problem such as sciatica, leaning over the sink to wash your face or brush your teeth can be extremely difficult and painful. To take strain off your lower back, place one foot on a stool or box. If this is not possible, keep your feet shoulder-width apart, bend your knees slightly, and lean forward at the hip. Try to keep your back straight.

HOW DOES THE TRAGER APPROACH TREAT SCIATICA?

The Trager approach combines physical and psychological treatment. A primary goal of the Trager approach is to break up those physiological and psychological patterns that cause pain and inhibit free movement of the spine. The practitioner applies gentle rotational movements with traction—a process of pulling and gently stretching muscles of the body—to the neck, legs, abdomen, back, and shoulders, and then rhythmically rocks each part of the body, in order to communicate a sense of how light, free, and easy movement can be.

As you experience the gentle and soothing movements of the Trager approach, the nerves that control muscle movement use this new information to recognize and release patterns of tension, pain, and muscle restriction. Rocking also promotes deep relaxation, so that muscular tension is further released on an emotional level. The psychological-physiological patterns are changed through the combination of joint mobilization, relaxation, and movement re-education. The result is the joining of body and mind for pain relief and overall well-being.

Practitioners of the Trager approach also teach simple movements, called *mentastics*, for clients to do at home. Mentastics are designed to recreate the feelings experienced during the Trager session and to build on the benefits of the session. The effects of mentastics include an increased sense of well-being, heightened levels of energy and vitality, greater mobility, and a renewed capacity for relaxation.

IS THERE CURRENT RELEVANT RESEARCH?

There are no specific research studies on the effectiveness of the Trager approach for the relief of sciatica. Moreover, in general, the scientific studies on the beneficial effects of Trager are limited. The field of Trager is in need of studies that follow standard research protocol in order to validate its effectiveness for a variety of conditions, including sciatica.

WHAT IS THE ESTIMATED COST AND DURATION
OF TREATMENT?

Generally, a Trager sessions costs $50 to $70 and lasts 60 to 90 minutes. A one-time session may helpful in relieving an acute attack. However, if you suffer from chronic sciatica problems, you will benefit most from repeated sessions and a commitment to at-home exercises.

IS MY HEALTH INSURANCE LIKELY TO COVER
THIS TREATMENT?

It is unlikely that the Trager approach is covered under your health plan. However, if your health plan covers some form of complementary medicine, it would be best to contact the person in charge of the complementary medicine portion of the policy and speak to him or her directly regarding the specifics of coverage. Also, it is possible that your health plan covers complementary medicine and you are not aware of it. In either case, contacting your health-plan organization and speaking to a knowledgeable representative would yield the best results.

WHAT PROFESSIONAL ORGANIZATION CAN I CONTACT FOR FURTHER INFORMATION?

The Trager Institute
21 Locust Avenue
Mill Valley, CA 94941
(415) 388–2688

IS THERE AN AT-HOME TECHNIQUE THAT I CAN USE?

Here is a simple at-home exercise that serves as an example of mentastics: when walking, before lowering your foot to the ground, shake your foot lightly as if you are trying to remove something stuck to the bottom of your shoe. You can feel how the rocking movement provides subtle comfort.

Conclusion

There are no hopeless situations; there are only people who have grown hopeless about them.

—Claire Booth Luce

Sciatica is a painful and often discouraging condition. Complementary medicine, in combination with conventional medicine, offers a magnified opportunity to maintain hope and to attain relief from sciatica's disturbing effects. By identifying your pain as sciatica and understanding its causes and symptoms, you are provided with the chance to reflect on your present lifestyle and to consider changes that will assist you in physical and emotional healing.

Treatments for the relief of sciatica are most effective when combined to create a comprehensive program that includes: specific therapeutic approaches integrated from both the conventional and complementary medicine fields; a modification in the activities of daily living that contribute to the condition; and stress management and/or relaxation. By blending the wisdom of complementary and conventional medicines, we are more likely to enhance our health and enact the healing process.

In researching this book, we have tried to include a balanced array of complementary approaches for the relief of sciatica. It was our intent to be as objective as possible in choosing applicable complementary approaches. We did not start this book with any preconceived biases, except for our commitment to the beneficial partnership that can be achieved between complementary and conventional medicine. To help us in bringing you the most helpful information through future projects, we would welcome your comments and feedback on this book. You can reach us through Avery Publishing Group or at the Endeavors Wellness Consulting Group.

Avery Publishing Group
Phone: (800) 548–5757
Website: www.averypublishing.com
E-mail: editors@averypublishing.com

Endeavors Wellness Consulting Group
Phone: (617) 489–4803
Fax: (617) 484–2756

Glossary

chi. A traditional Chinese medical term for the healing energy (or universal life energy) that circulates throughout the body.

chronic disorder. A long-term physical or emotional condition, usually with a slow-developing onset and often lasting for life, that is either persistently active or recurs frequently.

coccyx. A triangular-shaped bone that makes up the very end of the spinal column. It is formed from several rudimentary vertebrae.

complementary medicine. A term used to describe holistic (or wholistic) healing approaches that support and work in partnership with conventional medicine.

endorphins. Brain chemicals that serve as the body's natural opiates or pain killers.

holistic health. A philosophy of healing that takes into consideration aspects of the whole person—physical, emotional, mental, spiritual, social, and environmental factors. Holistic (or wholistic) health emphasizes the individual's active involvement in his or her own healthcare.

intervertebral discs. Composed of cartilage and also referred to simply as discs, these are parts of the spinal column that separate the vertebrae and cushion them during movement.

lymph. A body fluid that functions to remove foreign matter and toxins from the cell environment, transport necessary substances, and restore proper fluid content.

manipulation. The movement and adjustment of the joints and soft tissue of the body.

meridians. The specific pathways along which *chi*, or life energy, flows throughout the body. This concept is essential to Traditional Chinese Medicine techniques.

neuromuscular system. A term referring to the nerves and muscles of the body.

obstruction. A blockage or obstacle.

repressed emotions. Painful and / or stressful experiences and feelings that have been pushed into the unconscious mind and out of conscious awareness. The body represses emotions as a defense mechanism.

sacrum. Almost at the very end of the spinal column, this triangular-shaped bone plate is formed from five fused vertebrae. It is from behind the sacrum that the sciatic nerve originates.

sciatic nerve. A nerve, formed from several spinal nerves, that passes through the openings in the sacrum—the lower portion of the spine. It is the primary nerve in the leg, and the longest and largest nerve in the body. After originating in the low back, the sciatic nerve passes through the deep layers of the buttock muscles, through the back of the thigh, and sometimes as far down as the toes.

sciatica. An irritation or compression of the sciatic nerve. As a result of this condition, a sharp, electrical wave of pain, along with other symptoms such as numbness, tingling, weakness, achiness, and burning, can occur anywhere along the pathway of the sciatic nerve.

soft tissue. A term that refers to the muscles, tendons, ligaments, and organs of the body.

spinal cord. The bundle of nerves that stem from the brain and travel down the spinal canal, branching off at various areas to provide information and sensation to the body parts.

stressor. Any demand that causes an individual to feel overwhelmed and / or anxious. A stressor can be internal, such as an emotional hurt after a fight, or external, such as rush-hour traffic.

vertebrae. Twenty-four nearly circular-shaped bones that form an interlocking series, giving structure and strength to the spinal column. These bones protect the spinal cord and provide a vertical canal through which the cord can run. Channels in the vertebrae allow the various spinal nerves to branch off to their designated body parts.

Research Issues

In preparing to write this book, we decided it would be important to include research information on each discussed approach. But as evident throughout several of the sections, research studies unfortunately have not been conducted for all the approaches as they relate to sciatica. For this reason, we feel it is important to present a general overview on the state of research for complementary medicine.

THE NATIONAL CENTER FOR COMPLEMENTARY AND ALTERNATIVE MEDICINE (NCCAM)

In order to scientifically document the efficacy of complementary medicine, the Office of Alternative Medicine (OAM) was established in 1992 under the auspices of the National Institutes of Health (NIH). In 1998, the office was upgraded to the National Center for Complementary and Alternative Medicine (NCCAM). The Congressional mandate to the NCCAM states that its purpose is to "facilitate the evaluation of alternative medical treatment modalities to determine their effectiveness."

The NCCAM has now funded forty-two pilot research projects across the country, and has established eleven Specialty Research Centers to study complementary and alternative treatments for specific health conditions. The NCCAM does not act as a referral agency for complementary medicine treatments or practitioners, but it does disseminate information on complementary medicine to the public. The future goal of the NCCAM is to establish a comprehensive, electronic, bibliographic database of the scientific literature on complementary and alternative medical practices.[1]

RESEARCH APPROACHES

There are many factors influencing the state of research for complementary medicine. Among these are issues concerning inadequate funding; complementary medicine practitioners with little or no experience in research; and continued opposition from those who have a clear bias against complementary medicine. The major difficulty with the state of research, however, is in the research protocol.

Research has been conducted for years on numerous approaches of complementary medicine. Acupuncture, in particular, is very well studied. It is not the number of studies conducted that is in question, but the method of this research and its conformance to conventional trials. First, we will describe the general avenues of conventional medicine's research, and then elaborate on how complementary medicine can work with these patterns.

Research and Conventional Medicine

In conventional research studies, researchers are generally trying to identify the scientific basis for the specific action of a treatment process. For instance, in a drug study, researchers seek to isolate the active ingredient that brings about positive physical changes. However, in any treatment procedure, a number of different factors affect the outcome of the treatment process. These include the study participants' psychological and social influences, attitudes, and beliefs.

Obviously, these influences, attitudes, and beliefs cannot be measured in terms of the specific action they incur in the healing process. So they are often included under the umbrella term, "placebo effect." They are also regarded as "incidental" or "non-specific" treatment ingredients. Researchers take this into account when conducting studies. They create scenarios where the placebo factors can be isolated.

For example, let's take the case of researching a drug in order to observe the effects of an active ingredient. Researchers would randomly supply the drug to some of the study's participants, while the remainder would receive a similar-looking treatment that has no active ingredients. Assuming that all humans bring to the study their own "placebo" ingredients (attitudes, beliefs, etc.), the study is able to pinpoint the benefit of the drug used in the treatment process. Put into very simplified terms, if subjects in both groups experience similar benefits or disadvantages, it is likely that the drug is no more powerful than the placebo. But if the group on the drug attains different and more numerous benefits, it is likely that the medication is effective.

In the above scenario, if the researchers are aware of which participants are receiving the drug and which are receiving the placebo, the study is called a *randomized controlled study*. The participants are not informed whether they are receiving the active or the inactive substance in such a situation. And if neither the participants nor the practitioners know who is receiving the treatment and who is getting the placebo, the study is called a *randomized double-blind study*. These are the preferred methods of study for researchers today.

Research and Complementary Medicine

Due to its philosophy of taking an individualized approach to each person, complementary medicine has a difficult time fitting into the preferred research model described in the previous section. Practitioners consider the whole person (body, mind, and spirit) in designing a treatment plan, as well as lifestyle and dietary habits. Clients are also encouraged to become active participants in the treatment process. These philosophies and methods are critical to effective treatment in complementary medicine and are not easily eliminated for research purposes.

In terms of the approaches themselves, many complementary medicine treatments cannot be studied using a placebo. For example, with massage, it would be difficult to hide from participants that they were not actually receiving a massage treatment. And it would be almost impossible to set up a double-blind scenario where the practitioner is unaware of whether he or she is delivering the actual massage treatment.

In the case of acupuncture, advances have been made in research protocols, as well as isolating the scientific basis for positive outcomes. For instance, although there is no scientific proof that meridians exist, there is proof that an acupuncture treatment does release the pain-killing hormones called *endorphins* and *enkephalins*.[2] Attempts have been made to set up placebo controls by using what has been referred to as "sham acupuncture"—the practitioner places the needles on the body in locations other than the classical acupuncture points. Even with sham acupuncture, however, residual analgesic (pain-killing) effects result from the treatments. Therefore, studies are now being conducted with sham acupuncture where needle insertion is made only on the skin surface and not to the depth of effective acupuncture insertion, successfully eliminating even the residual effects.[3]

Aside from all the emphasis being placed on research protocol in order for complementary medicine to be considered effective, it should be noted that approximately only 15 percent of conventional medical treatments are supported by solid scientific evidence.[4] In fact, there are conventional medical treatments used today that have simply been handed down from generation to generation. These facts do not erase the need to provide the public, medical providers, and third-party payers with evidence on the efficacy of complementary medicine. As pointed out in Vincent and Furnham's *Complementary Medicine, A Research Perspective*, ". . . the difference in the standards of evidence for orthodox and complementary therapies may not be as great as generally assumed. There are certainly, as we shall see, many flaws in studies of complementary medicine. However, in the face of similar problems with the evidence for orthodox medicine, it is unreasonable, even hypocritical, for critics of complementary medicine to throw up their hands in horror, dismissing the existing studies out of hand."

How then does complementary medicine provide research to satisfy the conventional medical community? The answer lies with continued perseverance to develop ongoing, effective, and valid studies that are evaluated and designed in collaboration with respected research and medical professionals in both the complementary and conventional communities. The debate on research methods and the differences in approaches between conventional and complementary medicine will continue. The good news is that through debate and the understanding of these differences, researchers will be able to determine the most effective ways in which to scientifically study complementary medicine. What we will see in the future is a new model of health care that incorporates the philosophy of complementary medicine into scientific research.

Health Insurance Issues

Insurance coverage for complementary medicine is an ever-changing subject. But to help you familiarize yourself with some of the issues involved, the following pages will provide up-to-date information on the broad trends in the area of insurance coverage for complementary care. We also project a little into the future, considering what is possible and what may happen as the demand for complementary treatments increases. For treatment-specific information, see the individual approach sections; we make general statements whether or not the approach, according to our research, is covered in some form by insurance. It is not appropriate to list individual companies and their policies, as the industry is constantly changing.

INCREASES IN COVERAGE

Not long ago, insurance coverage for complementary medicine was sparse. Yet within even the past couple of years, there has been an incredible jump in the number of insurance companies covering some form of complementary medicine. In 1996, eighteen large insurance and managed-care companies either had policies in place to cover complementary medicine, or were developing policies to do so.

According to a survey conducted by Decision Resources in 1995, 86 percent of the largest HMOs in the country cover some type of complementary medicine.[1] Today, there are thirty major insurers covering more than one complementary medicine approach.[2] Why is there such an increase in coverage for complementary medicine? The answer lies in two major reasons: consumer demand and potential cost savings.

Consumer Demand

With increased patient demand, insurance companies are becoming more competitive, striving to increase and/or maintain enrollment. A 1998 survey titled Landmark Report I on Public Perceptions of Alternative Care reported, "45 percent of people polled would be willing to pay each month to have access to alternative care, and 67 percent said the availability of an alternative healthcare component was an important consideration in choosing a health plan."[3] The 1999 Landmark Report II on HMOs and Alternative Care shows that nearly three-fourths of HMOs (or 74 percent) believe consumer demand for complementary care will be moderate or strong in the future.[4] Insurance companies are, therefore, responding to the market demand for complementary medicine.

Potential Cost Savings

Proponents of complementary medicine believe that treatment costs for complementary care will be significantly lower than conventional medical treatment. This has been proven for chiropractic care; RAND Corporation published a large study in 1990 that found chiropractors were more successful at treating patients with chronic, low back pain and that chiropractic care was about one-tenth the cost of conventional care.[5] But it remains unknown whether long-term savings result from using other complementary medicine procedures. Insurance companies are also having a difficult time in establishing exact costs and duration of treatment for complementary care.

An additional factor related to cost savings is the issue of initial marketing fees—that is, comparing these fees with estimated long-term savings. Those who claim that coverage for complementary medicine treatments will incur lower costs may not be taking into account the amount of money companies need to spend to market their coverage of these services. Simply offering complementary medicine services as a rider to existing policies does not guarantee that employers will buy into them for their employees. This means that insurance companies may need to spend more money marketing to individuals and businesses. Also, because complementary medicine coverage is so new to the industry, there are no long-term statistics on cost savings for the insurance companies. Some insurance companies and HMOs may find that the wait is not worth the amount of money they are spending.

AVAILABLE TYPES OF COVERAGE

The type of coverage provided by insurance companies is quite varied. These differences have to do with the insurance companies themselves deciding the type and quantity of coverage, and diverse state mandates requiring coverage. For example, in more than forty states, it is mandated that chiropractic care be covered by health insurance. However, some type of insurance coverage exists for chiropractic care in all fifty states.

There are ways of getting around state mandates too. For example, in Nevada, all health insurance companies are required to cover acupuncture. However, some employer-sponsored insurance programs are not regulated by the state. Therefore, even though there may be a state mandate to cover an approach, not all individuals will benefit.

Here's an example of yet another complication to consider. Because Blue Cross and Blue Shield of Pennsylvania operates as a managed services plan, the state legislature dictates who the acceptable providers are. Presently, the only complementary medicine practitioners recognized by this legislation are chiropractors. Some companies may offer services for complementary medicine through a rider to existing policies, while others offer direct access through a network of screened complementary health practitioners. So coverage varies greatly, according to the insurance company.

Contrary to the general perception, coverage for complementary medicine is, quite often, not based on prevention. And similar to conventional medicine, coverage can be dependent on a particular diagnosis, and set for an allotted number of visits or for a dollar amount.

THE DIRECTION OF COVERAGE

The direction of health insurance coverage for complementary medicine will continue to evolve. Coverage for some approaches may be added or expanded as they are proven effective in peer-reviewed medical literature, or mandated by state law. Some may be dropped if proven ineffective. Some companies have already had to drop coverage for certain procedures, due to the inability to estimate and control utilization. The overall consensus is that consumers will continue to play the lead role in determining coverage for complementary medicine. Employers and individuals will continue to have an impact on insurance companies' decisions to add or expand complementary medicine coverage.

In past years, coverage for complementary medicine was prevalent only in the western part of the country. Now, however, the coverage is spreading across the country. In the northeast, where coverage was once scant, a major insurer with over 1.5 million members now has the largest network (over 2,000) of complementary medicine practitioners available through direct access.[6] Chiropractic care, osteopathy, and acupuncture are the three approaches most widely covered by insurance, but once again, the coverage will vary from company to company and from state to state.[7]

Some companies will review coverage on a case by case basis. Also, there are companies presently covering some complementary medicine approaches but that are not advertising it. You will have to contact your insurance company to get the specifics on treatment coverage. Inquire about present coverage and the possibility of future coverage of complementary medicine. With persistence, you may be able to encourage an employer to purchase the additional rider for complementary medicine. Or maybe you will persuade your insurance company to pay for complementary medicine treatments even if it does not cover complementary medicine for your regular policy. The more that customers inquire and request, the greater the chance for insurance companies to respond to the movement toward comprehensive coverage that includes complementary medicine.

Notes

Preface

1. American Physical Therapy Association, "Low back pain," *APTA Fact Sheet* (Alexandria, VA: American Physical Therapy Association, 1997).

2. Clayton L Thomas, M.D., M.P.H., ed, *Tabor's Cyclopedic Medical Dictionary* (Philadelphia, PA: F.A. Davis Company, 1993).

3. American Chiropractic Association, *Manipulation for my back problem? An informative guide outlining the benefits of manipulation for back problems* (Arlington, VA: American Chiropractic Association, 1995).

4. J Frymoyer, "Back pain and sciatica," *New England Journal of Medicine* 318(5) (1988): 291–300, cited in Cheryl Cummings Stegbauer, Ph.D., C.F.N.C., "Sciatic pain and piriformis syndrome," *The Nurse Practitioner* 22(5) (May 1997): 166–180.

5. American Physical Therapy Association, "Low back pain," *APTA Fact Sheet* (Alexandria, VA: American Physical Therapy Association, 1997).

6. Frymoyer, *New England Journal of Medicine*, 291–300.

7. American Physical Therapy Association. "Low back pain," *APTA Fact Sheet* (Alexandria, VA: American Physical Therapy Association, 1997).

8. Frymoyer, *New England Journal of Medicine*, 291–300.

PART I

Defining Sciatica

1. P Barton, "Piriformis syndrome: A rational approach to management," *Pain* 47 (1991): 345–352.

2. Associated Press. "Researchers eye mutant gene as the cause of some back pain," *Boston Herald*, (July 17, 1999): 13.

Treating Sciatica

1. JT Cottingham, and J Maitland, "A three-paradigm treatment model using soft tissue mobilization and guided movement-awareness techniques for a patient with chronic low back pain: a case study," *Journal of Orthopedic Sports Physical Therapy* 26(3) (1997): 155–167.

2. JW Vlaeyen, et al., "Behavioral rehabilitation of chronic low back pain," *British Journal of Clinical Psychology* 34(1) (Feb 1995): 95–118.

3. JS Kriegler, and Z.S. Ashenberg, "Management of chronic low back pain: a comprehensive approach," *Seminar of Neurology* 7(4) (Dec 1987): 303–312.

4. DM Eisenberg, et al., "Trends in alternative medicine use in the United States, 1990–1997: results of a follow-up national study," *Journal of the American Medical Association* 280 (1998): 1569–1575.

5. Eisenberg, et al., *Journal of the American Medical Association*, 1569–1575.

6. Eisenberg, et al., *Journal of the American Medical Association*, 1569–1575.

7. Eisenberg, et al., *Journal of the American Medical Association*, 1569–1575.

8. Eisenberg, et al., *Journal of the American Medical Association*, 1569–1575.

9. Eisenberg, et al., *Journal of the American Medical Association*, 1569–1575.

10. MS Wetzel, DM Eisenberg, and TJ Kaptchuk, "Courses involving complementary and alternative medicine at US medical schools," *Journal of the American Medical Association* 280 (1998): 784–787.

11. Jeanne Achterberg, Ph.D., "Between lightning and thunder: the pause before the shifting paradigm," *Alternative Therapies* 4(3) (May 1998): 62–66.

12. Phil B Fontanarosa, M.D., and George D Lundberg, M.D., "Complementary, alternative, unconventional, and integrative medicine," *Journal of the American Medical Association* 278(23) (Dec 17, 1997): 2111–2112.

13. Clayton L Thomas, M.D., M.P.H., ed, *Tabor's Cyclopedic Medical Dictionary* (Philadelphia, PA: F.A. Davis Company, 1993).

14. Carol Lewis, "What to do when your back is in pain," *FDA Consumer* 32(2) (Mar/Apr 1998): 26(4).

15. JT Cottingham, and J Maitland, *Journal of Orthopedic Sports Physical Therapy*, 155–167.

PART II

Acupuncture

1. National Institutes of Health. *Consensus Development Statement, Acupuncture* (Bethesda, MD: National Institutes of Health, Nov 3–5, 1997).

Alexander Technique

1. O Elkayam, et al., "Multidisciplinary approach to chronic back pain: prognostic elements of the outcome," *Clinical Experimental Rheumatology* 14(3) (May/Jun 1996): 281–288.

2. Keren Fisher, "Early experiences of a multidisciplinary pain management programme," *Holistic Medicine* 3(1) (1988): 47–56.

Aquatic Therapy

1. Joanne M Koury, *Aquatic Therapy Programming* (Champaign, IL: Human Kinetics, 1996).

2. SR Vickery, KJ Cureton, and JL Langstaff, "Heart rate and energy expenditure during Aqua Dynamics," *The Physician and Sports Medicine* 11(3) (1983): 67–72.

3. T Heberlein, et al., "The metabolic cost of high impact and hydroaerobic exercise in middle-aged females," unpublished research from the Department of Physical Education, Adelphi University, Garden City, NY, 1989.

Chiropractic

1. PG Shekelle, et al., "Spinal manipulation for low-back pain," *Annals of Internal Medicine* 117 (1992): 590–598.

2. WJ Assendelft, et al., "The efficacy of chiropractic manipulation for back pain: blinded review of relevant randomized clinical trials," *Journal of Manipulative Physiological Therapies* 15(8) (Oct 1992): 487–494.

3. S Bigos, et al., *Acute Low Back Problems in Adults: Clinical Practice Guidelines* (No. 14), (Rockville, Md: Agency for Health Care Policy

and Research, Public Health Service, U.S. Department of Health and Human Services, Dec 1994), AHCPR publication 0642.

4. BW Koes, et al., "Spinal manipulation for low back pain: An updated systematic review of randomized clinical trials," *Spine* 21(24) (1996): 2860–2871.

5. ID Coulter, "Efficacy and Risks of Chiropractic Manipulation: What Does the Evidence Suggest?" *Integrative Medicine* 1 (1998): 61–66.

6. TF Bergmann, and BV Jongeward, "Manipulative therapy in lower back pain with leg pain and neurological deficit," *Journal of Manipulative Physiological Therapies* 21 (May 1998): 4, 288–294.

Emotional Pain Relief Therapy

1. John E Sarno, *Healing Back Pain* (New York, NY: Warner Books, 1991).

2. John E Sarno, *The Mindbody Prescription* (New York, NY: Warner Books, 1998).

3. Benson, Herbert, and Eileen M Stuart, *The Wellness Book* (New York, NY: Simon and Schuster, 1993) p. 12.

Foot Reflexology

1. Wang Liang, "An exploration of the clinical indications of foot reflexology—a retrospective of its clinical application to 8,096 cases," *Reflexions* (Winter / Spring 1997): 3–6.

Hatha Yoga

1. R LaForge, "Mind-body fitness: encouraging prospects for primary and secondary prevention," *Journal Cardiovascular Nursing* 11(3) (1997): 53–65.

Massage

1. Tiffany Fields, Ph.D., Touch Research Institute, University of Miami School of Medicine, "Research at TRI," *The Touch Research Institute,* www.miami.edu / touch-research, (1999). (Phone: 305–243–6781)

Myotherapy

1. Tiffany Fields, Ph.D., Touch Research Institute, University of Miami School of Medicine, "Research at TRI," *The Touch Research Institute,* www.miami.edu / touch-research, (1999). (Phone: 305–243–6781)

Nutritional Counseling

1. *The Back Letter* 11(7) (Jul 1996): 77(1).

2. James F Balch, M.D., and Phyllis A Balch, C.N.C., *Prescription for Nutritional Healing* (Second Edition) (Garden City Park, NY: Avery Publishing Group, 1996).

Osteopathy

1. Ernst E Pittler, "Experts' opinions on complementary/alternative therapies for low back pain," *Journal of Manipulative Physiological Therapy* 22(2) (Feb, 1999): 87–90.

Personal Training

1. BW Nelson, et al., "The clinical effects of intensive, specific exercise on chronic low back pain: a controlled study of 895 consecutive patients with 1-year follow up," *Orthopedics* 10 (Oct 18, 1995): 971–981.

2. Miriam Nelson, "Staying Strong," *Tuftonia* (Spring 1997): 12–18.

3. National Institutes of Health, "Physical Activity and Cardiovascular Health—NIH Consensus Panel," *Journal of the American Medical Association* 276(3) (Jul 17, 1996).

Qigong

1. Kenneth M Sancier, "Medical Applications of Qigong," *Alternative Therapies* 2(1) (Jan 1996): 40–46.

Relaxation/Meditation

1. "Integration of behavioral and relaxation approaches into the treatment of chronic pain and insomnia," *Journal of the American Medical Association* 276(4) (Jul 24/31, 1996): 313–318.

Rolfing

1. Valerie Hunt, and Wayne Mansey, UCLA Department of Kinesiology, "Research on Rolfing," *The Rolf Institute,* www.rolf.org, (1999).

2. JT Cottingham, et al., "Shifts in pelvic inclination angle and parasympathetic tone produced by Rolfing soft tissue manipulation," *Physical Therapy* 68(9) (Sep 1988): 1364–1370.

3. "Bodywork methods relieve chronic low back pain," *Massage Magazine* 71 (Feb, 1998): 21.

Tai Chi

1. TI Bhatti, et al., "Tai chi as a treatment for chronic low back pain: a randomized, controlled study," *Alternative Therapies in Health and Medicine* 4(2) (Mar 1998): 90.

Research Issues

1. National Institutes of Health, Office of Alternative Medicine Clearinghouse, *General Information Package* (Bethesda, MD: National Institutes of Health, Mar 1997).

2. Charles Vincent, and Adrian Furnham, *Complementary Medicine, A Research Perspective* (West Sussex, England: John Wiley and Sons, Ltd., 1997).

3. Charles Vincent, and Adrian Furnham, *Complementary Medicine, A Research Perspective.*

4. Charles Vincent, and Adrian Furnham, *Complementary Medicine, A Research Perspective.*

Health Insurance Issues

1. Jan Goodwin, "A Health Insurance Revolution," *New Age Journal* (Mar / Apr 1997): 95–99.

2. Robert Cunningham, ed., "Expanding Coverage Signals Growing Demand, Acceptance for Alternative Care," *Medicine & Health Perspectives* (New York, NY: Faulkner and Gray's Healthcare Information Center, May 4, 1998), p. 1–4.

3. *Alternative Therapies in Health and Medicine* 4(2) (Mar 1998).

4. Landmark Healthcare, *1999 Landmark Report II on HMOs and Alternative Care,* www.landmarkhealthcare.com / research.htm, (May 1999).

5. "News Briefs," *American Journal of Health Promotion* 12(2).

6. Interview with Beverly Schuch, CNNF Anchor, and Dr. Hassan Rifaat, Director, Oxford Health Alternative Medicine Department, *Take It Personally,* CNNF, July 28, 1997.

7. Jan Goodwin, *New Age Journal,* 95–99.

Index

Acupressure, 27–30
Acupuncture, 30–34
Alexander technique, 34–38
Alternative medicine. See
   Complementary medicine.
American Academy of Pastoral
   Counselors, 54, 99
American Association of Nutritional
   Consultants, 79
American Board of Hypnotherapy,
   100
American Chiropractic Association, 46
American College for Advancement
   in Medicine, 79, 84
American Council on Exercise, 88
American Dietetic Association, 79
American Massage Therapy
   Association, 69
American Medical Association Archives,
   19
American Oriental Bodywork
   Therapy Association, 30, 93, 108
American Osteopathic Association, 82
American Psychiatric Association, 54,
   100
American Psychological Association,
   54, 100
American Society of Clinical
   Hypothesis, 100
Ankylosing spondylitis, 13
Aquatic Exercise Association, 42
Aquatic therapy, 38–42
Aromatherapy, 70
Artemisia vulgaris, 32
Arthritis, 12–13

Association for Applied Psychophysiology and Biofeedback, 100
Awareness Through Movement, 55

Back pain. *See* Sciatica.
Bicycling, 89
Bioenergetics, 48
Biofeedback, 95
Biofeedback Certification Institute
   of America, 100
Bonnie Prudden Pain Erasure, 74

Cat stretch, 64
Chi, 27, 30, 90, 105
Chiropractic, 42–46
Christian meditation, 95
Coccyx, 3
Cognitive restructuring, 48
Complementary medicine
   approach of, 17–21
   issues to consider, concerning,
     20–21
   research and, 19, 119–120
   selecting types of, 20
   trends for use of, 18–19
Complementary Medicine, A Research
   Perspective, 120
Connective tissue, 4
Contemplation, 95
Conventional medicine, 15–17
   research and, 118–119
Core energetics, 49
Cortisol, 94
Craniosacral therapy, 83
Cross fiber friction massage, 67
Cupping, 32

Deep pressure massage. *See*
     Myotherapy.
Degenerative arthritis. *See*
     Osteoarthritis.

Electro-acupuncture, 32
Emotional pain relief therapy, 46–54
Emotional stress, 11–12
Endometrial cysts, 13
Endometriosis, 13
Endorphins, 119
Enkephalins, 119
Epinephrine, 94
Exercise program, developing. *See*
     Personal training.

Feldenkrais Guild, 57
Feldenkrais method, 55–57
Fields, Tiffany, 68, 72
Foot reflexology, 58–61
Functional Integration, 55

Genetic research, 11
Gestalt therapy, 49
Ginger, 32
Golf, 88
Guided imagery, 49, 95

Hatha yoga, 61–65
Health insurance
     consumer demands and, 122
     cost savings, potential and, 122
     coverage, available types of, 123
     coverage, direction of, 123–124
     increases in coverage and, 121
Heat therapy. *See* Moxibustion.
Hydrotherapy, 41
Hypnotherapy, 95–96

Integrative Medicine, 44
International Association of Yoga
     Therapists, 64
International Institute of Reflexology,
     61
Internation Myotherapy Association,
     74
Invertebral discs, 3

*Journal of Manipulative Physiological
     Therapy,* 81

*Journal of Orthopedic and Sports
     Physical Therapy,* 22, 103
*Journal of the American Medical
     Association,* 19

Lactic acid, 94
Laser acupuncture, 32
Ligaments, 4
Lillo, Robert A., 77
Low back pain, 6
Lumbar discs, 8–9
Lumbar herniated disc, 8–9
Lumbosacral muscle strain, 9–10

Massage, 65–70
Massage Magazine, 103
Medication, 16
Meditation. *See* Relaxation/
     Meditation.
Mentastics, 110
Meridians, 27, 30, 90
Moxa, 32
Moxibustion, 32
Mugwort, 32
Muscles, 4, 14
Myotherapy, 71–75

National Acupuncture and Oriental
     Medicine Alliance, 34
National Association of Social
     Workers, 54, 100
National Center for Complementary
     and Alternative Medicine
     (NCCAM), 117
National Certification Board for
     Therapeutic Massage and
     Bodywork, 70
National Guild of Hypnotists, 101
NCCAM. *See* National Center for
     Complementary and Alternative
     Medicine.
Nerves, 3
Neurolinguistic programming (NLP),
     50
NLP. *See* Neurolinguistic
     programming.
Nonsteroidal anti-inflammatory
     drugs (NSAIDs), 15, 16

North American Society of Teachers of the Alexander Technique, 38
NSAIDs. *See* Nonsteroidal anti-inflammatory drugs.
Nutritional counseling, 75–80
Nutritional recommendations, 79–80

Orthopedics, 86
Osteoarthritis, 12
Osteopathy, 80–82, 84

Personal training, 84–90
Physical therapy, 16–17
Piriformis muscles, 8
Piriformis syndrome, 8
Posture habits, poor, eliminating. *See* Alexander technique.
Prescription for Nutritional Healing (Balch and Balch), 79
Progressive muscle relaxation, 96
Proprioceptive neuromuscular facilitation (PNF), 17, 67
Psychophysiological interactions, 52
Psychotherapy. *See* Emotional pain relief therapy.

Qigong, 90–93

Relaxation/Meditation, 93–101
Research issues, 117–120
Rheumatoid arthritis, 12
Rolf Institute, 105
Rolfing, 101–105
Running, 89
Ruptured disc, 10–11

Sacroiliac ligament tear, 13–14
Sacrum, 3, 5, 13
Sarno, John E., 47, 51
Sciatic nerve, 5
    causes of irritation of, 7–14
Sciatica
    about, 3–7
    causes of, 7–14
    genetics and, 11
    symptoms of, 7
    treating, 15–22
Science, 11

Shields, Robert, 22
Siddha meditation, 96
Skiing, 89
Spinal canal, 10
Spinal cord, 3
Spinal stenosis, 10
Spondylitis, 13
Sports massage, 66
Stress, coping with. *See* Relaxation/Meditation.
Stress management, 50, 96
Stressors, types of, 11
Stretches, 74–75
Surgery, 17
Swedish massage, 67
Swimming, 89

Tai chi, 105–108
TCM. *See* Traditional Chinese medicine.
Tendons, 4
Tennis, 88–89
TENS. *See* Transcutaneous electrical nerve stimulation.
Tension myositis syndrome (TMS), 47, 51
TMS. *See* Tension myositis syndrome.
Traction, 17
Traditional Chinese medicine (TCM), 27
Trager approach, 108–111
Trager Institute, the, 111
Transcendental meditation, 96–97
Transcendental Meditation, 101
Transcutaneous electrical nerve stimulation (TENS), 16–17

Ultrasound, 17
Using anchors, 50

Vertebrae, 3, 4
Visualization, 49

Water therapy. *See* Aquatic therapy.
Weight lifting, 89
Wellness Book, The, (Benson and Stuart), 50

Everything You Need to Know About Choosing An
Effective Complementary Healthcare Treatment

Your Guide to
Complementary
MEDICINE

Includes Naturopathy, Acupuncture, Holistic
Dentistry, Shiatsu,
Herbal Medicine,
Tai Chi, Massage,

Bodywork, Traditional Chinese Medicine, Yoga,
Reflexology, Ayurveda,
Acupressure, Homeopathy,
Biofeedback, Meditation,
Nutrition, Aromatherapy, and Much More

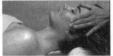

Larry P. Credit Sharon G. Hartunian Margaret J. Nowak

6" x 9" • 208 pages • ISBN 0-89529-831-7 • $10.95 U.S.